A Scientific Colloquium of the Department of Oto-Rhino-Laryngology,
University of Tübingen, January 24, 1987

Recent Concepts in ORL

Volume Editors
K. Jahnke, Tübingen
C.R. Pfaltz, Basel

53 figures, 5 color plates and 21 tables, 1988

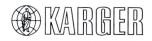

Basel · München · Paris · London · New York · New Delhi · Singapore · Tokyo · Sydney

Advances in Oto-Rhino-Laryngology

Cover illustration
Creation of a promontory window according to Plester, on the basis of anatomic studies.

Library of Congress Cataloging-in-Publication Data
Recent concepts in ORL: a scientific colloquium of the
Department of Oto-rhino-laryngology, University of Tübingen, January 24, 1987 /
volume editors, K. Jahnke, C. R. Pfaltz.
(Advances in oto-rhino-laryngology; vol. 39)
Symposium held in honour of Prof. Dr. Dietrich Plester
on the occasion of his 65th birthday.
Includes index.
ISBN 3–8055–4725–0
1. Otolaryngology-Congresses. 2. Plester, D.
I. Jahnke, Klaus. II. Pfaltz, C. R. (Carl Rudolf) III. Plester, D.
IV. Universitäts-Hals-Nasen-Ohrenklinik Tübingen. V. Series.
[DNLM: 1. Otorhinolaryngologic Diseases-congresses.
W1 AD701 v. 39/WV 100 R2955 1987]
RF 16.A38 vol. 39
617′.51-dc 19

Bibliographic Indices
This publication is listed in bibliographic services, including Current Contents® and Index Medicus.

Drug Dosage
The authors and the publisher have exerted every effort to ensure that drug selection and dosage set forth in this text are in accord with current recommendations and practice at the time of publication. However, in view of ongoing research, changes in government regulations, and the constant flow of information relating to drug therapy and drug reactions, the reader is urged to check the package insert for each drug for any change in indications and dosage and for added warnings and precautions. This is particularly important when the recommended agent is a new and/or infrequently employed drug.

© Copyright 1988 by S. Karger AG, P.O. Box, CH–4009 Basel (Switzerland)
Printed in Switzerland by Thür AG, Offsetdruck, Pratteln
ISBN 3–8055–4725–0

Recent Concepts in ORL

Advances in Oto-Rhino-Laryngology

Vol. 39

Series Editor
C.R. Pfaltz, Basel

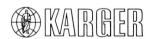 KARGER

Basel · München · Paris · London · New York · New Delhi · Singapore · Tokyo · Sydney

Contents

Preface

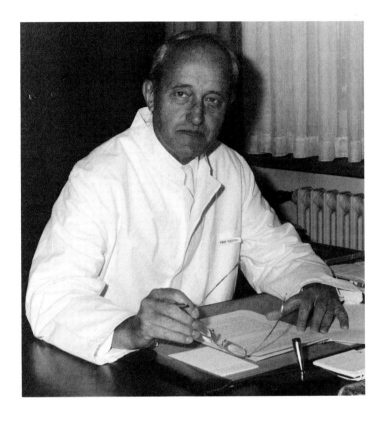

    Prof. Dietrich Plester, MD, was born in 1922 in Essen, Westfalia, where his schooling took place. After studying medicine at the universities of Würzburg and Berlin, he served in the military with an ensuing period as prisoner of war. Thereupon he received his academic research training at the Departments of Pathology and Pharmacology of the University of Düsseldorf, Medical School. During this time, he conducted experimental investigations into the action of pharmaceuticals on the autonomic nervous system. Between 1951 and 1954, he served as ENT resident under the guidance of Prof. H.L. Wullstein, who was then in Siegen, Westfalia. Since then his special attention has been focussed on the surgical improvement of hearing deficits. In 1955, he became first senior resident and later associate professor in the Department of Otorhinolaryngology of Düsseldorf, for Prof. Meyer zum Gottesberge, whose understanding and stimulating leadership made it possible to intensively take part in the tempestuous development of middle ear surgery. Soon a pioneer himself, Prof. Plester was honored on numerous occasions. He became a Honorable member of the British Royal Society of Medicine, as well as of Societies of Oto-Rhino-Laryngology on all continents. In addition he is a member of the Collegium otorhinolaryngologicum amicitiae sacrum and a member of the Leopoldina, Halle/Saale, the oldest German academy of nature sciences and medicine. Aside from his clinical and surgical activities, Prof. Plester conducted research into the metabolism of the inner ear with the use of radioisotopes. Between 1954 and 1963, he visited southern Sudan, together with Dr. Rosen and other colleagues from different countries, to study the hearing of native populations. Compared with data from populations of different life-styles (Egypt, Germany, USA), important conclusions as to the etiology and pathogenesis of presbyacusis could be made.

Prof. Dietrich Plester was installed as head of the Department of Otorhinolaryngology, University of Tübingen, in November 1966. Here he founded his own 'school' in otologic surgery. The hearing-impaired patient always remained in the foreground, and was treated with incomparable empathy and care. In this vein, and with outmost attention to surgical and technical detail, he trained many colleagues in the art of microsurgery of the ear. Together with them, to date he has conducted 20 courses on microsurgical technique in Tübingen, which were attended by nearly 1,000 ENT surgeons most of whom come from German-speaking countries. An even greater stream of visitors from the whole world denotes the immense influence Prof. Plester has gained by his operative demonstrations. This has made its mark on contemporary middle ear surgery. In addition, he has held many lectures and has written multiple publications, along with those of his students. His critizism has always been of outmost value in questions concerning clinical and research investigations. As impetus for histologic studies of the middle ear, the use of new biomaterials in reconstructive surgery and the immunology of the inner ear, he has played an important role. The same applies for other clinical aspects of our field, as in tumor, reconstructive plastic and emergency surgery, which he supported with his wide scientific and clinical experience. As a result, the contributions in this book offer a wide spectrum, and are presented in thanks from his students and friends for his decades of long activity as surgeon, teacher and scientist.

Klaus Jahnke

Foreword

At the end of January, 1987, a symposium was held at the University of Tübingen in honour of Prof. Dr. Dietrich Plester, chairman of the Department of Otorhinolaryngology, on the occasion of his 65th birthday. A symposium of this kind may become either a scientifically embellished distinction of the person who is celebrating his jubilee; or – as in the present case – it becomes a state-of-the-art review of the scientific and clinical progress in a medical field to which the honoured person has made substantial contributions during his active years as head of the department.

D. Plester belongs to the generation of ORL surgeons who – entering their specialty shortly after the war – have witnessed the enormous and rapid development of surgical management of ENT diseases, in particular microsurgery of the ear. In the early 1950s a hitherto inaccessible, vast dimension of surgery was opened, inaugurating a new era of surgical knowledge and treatment. With the advent of antibiotics ORL surgery became more and more function-orientated because preoperative infections could be cured and postoperative infective complications prevented. Reconstructive surgery of the middle ear became the primary goal; in cases of chronic otitis media and cholesteatoma not only could the disease be eradicated in the majority of cases but also auditory function preserved or even improved. In otosclerosis or malformations of the middle ear cleft it became possible to restore a socially adequate hearing. Moritz, Wullstein and Zoellner on the one hand and Lempert, Rosen, Shea and Portmann on the other, were some of the promotors of these new techniques, providing the fundamental knowledge which later became the solid basis for the further development of tympanoplasty, ossiculoplasty and stapedectomy.

D. Plester had the opportunity to experience at first hand the rapidly developing techniques of modern ear surgery. Rather soon he innovated his own methods and gradually became one of the leading personalities in this field. However, in contrast to other successful ear surgeons he never considered reconstructive surgery of the ear a merely technical problem. His academic background – basic training in pharmacology and physiology – had formed his scientific mind so strongly that – as a surgeon – he always considered the pathophysiological problem the most important one, determining the performance of his surgical technique. He never accepted or developed new methods – even if they became or were 'fashionable' at a certain period – which were not consistent with his strict prerequisites concerning the indication, the pathophysiological basis and the eventual short or longstanding risk of an operation. This may explain why he has been so successful.

As department head he felt not only responsible of the subspecialty of otology but of the whole field of oto-rhino-laryngology. This attitude is reflected by the various contributions made at the Tübingen Symposium by friends and pupils. They cover the whole field of ORL – from basic research in inner ear biology and physiology to laser surgery many important scientific and clinical problems are discussed. They will not only interest the clinician but also the practicing ENT specialist, according to the rules of Dietrich Plester's school that scientific activities should never become a performance of 'l'art pour l'art' but should always be clinically relevant.

C.R. Pfaltz

Laudatio

On the Occasion of the 65th Birthday of Prof. Plester, Tübingen

Adolf Miehlke, Göttingen

Ladies and Gentlemen,

rather than enumerating the vast number of Honorary Memberships of National ENT Societies held by Prof. Plester in about 90 countries, I shall go about my task in a different way.

Dietrich Plester was born January 23, 1922 in Essen. His birthplace is of importance since it lies in a former province of Prussia, called 'Westfalen'. This land stands for willpower, tenacity, firmness of attitude and other virtues which have become all but extinct nowadays in many persons of public standing. It was D. Plester's good fortune that Westfalen had become Prussian, imbuing him with basic principles that are increasingly acknowledged once again in both parts of Germany.

Genealogically the name Plester is derived from a mill, the socalled *Pleister mill* in southern Westfalen. No wonder he and I should become friends as my name, Miehlke, also derives from mill, meaning 'little mill'.

The idea of what Prussia stood for is being revived at both sides of the Iron Curtain, not the deprecatory, negative image of the 'bad junker' but the positive traits summarized as follows by Friedrich Christoph Dettinger (1702–1782): (1) Sense of duty; (2) loyalty; (3) pleasure in one's work for its own sake; (4) honesty of thinking; (5) devotion to the common welfare; (6) steadfastness.

I shall proceed to illustrate these traits as evidenced by Dietrich Plester's career.

(1) Duty: By faithfully serving in his various offices and in his attitude towards his patients and students, he has shown himself as an example of a person living for his duties.

(2) Loyalty: His former teacher, Prof. Meyer zum Gottesberge, is attesting D. Plester a high sense of loyalty of which he gave ample proof through the years of his apprenticeship and later on.

(3) Work for its own sake: An outline is given of the many scientific accomplishments in clinical medicine, especially in ENT but also in pharmacology. Moreover, as a young man he conducted important ethnographic studies, discovering a hitherto unknown African people, the Pre-Nilotes who live on the Upper Nile. This was not without danger as illustrated by his near fatal encounter with a most unscientifically-minded lion.

(4) Honest thinking: There is perfect frankness in the way he leads his clinic and discusses problems with his staff, with no immovable preformed opinions adhered to.

(5) Common welfare: In his truly international clinic he has given his unique professional skill to innumerable patients and strives to extend and spread his knowledge also for the benefit of his colleagues who come to learn from him in courses held in Tübingen and during demonstrations on all continents.

(6) Steadfastness: In his lifetime he has shown himself to be able to face and master the most difficult situations. He is a staunch friend as is his wife, Lore Plester.

Adv. Oto-Rhino-Laryng., vol. 39, pp. 1–12 (Karger, Basel 1988)

The Morphologic Basis for Perilymphatic Gushers and Oozers[1]

Harold F. Schuknecht[a], Christoph Reisser[b]

[a] Harvard Medical School, and [b] Department of Otolaryngology,
Massachusetts Eye and Ear Infirmary, Boston, Mass., USA

A disconcerting experience for the otologic surgeon is a sudden rush of perilymphatic fluid coincident with fenestrating or removing the footplate of the stapes. In clinical experience the phenomenon occurs only rarely in ears with normal cochlear function but much more frequently in ears having conductive and/or sensorineural hearing loss of congenital origin. There are numerous descriptions in the literature of spontaneous [1–12] and surgically induced [13–19] profuse perilymphatic fluid leaks from the oval windows of ears with congenital hearing losses. While the incidence of the condition as an occurrence during otologic surgery has not been documented, it occurs often enough to have generated the common parlance of 'gusher' [19] for a pouring, jet-like outflow and 'oozer' for a milder welling-type of flowage. Clearly, only the first milliliter or two are true perilymph fluid and the remainder is cerebrospinal fluid (CSF). In reference to gushers and oozers, the term perilymphatic is preferable to perilymph for it implies only that the fluid is emerging from the perilymphatic space. It is obvious that these ears have an abnormally large connection between the subarachnoid and perilymphatic spaces.

It has been assumed by most otologic surgeons that a widely patent cochlear aqueduct is the most probable site for such a confluence. Indeed,

[1] This work was supported by Grant 5 R01 NS05881 from the National Institute of Neurological and Communicative Disorders and Stroke.

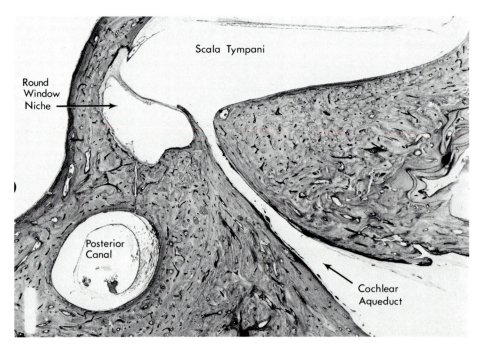

Fig. 1. Patent cochlear aqueduct of a 67-year-old man. At its narrowest point the lumen measures 0.2 mm in diameter.

temporal bone studies have shown that widely patent cochlear aqueducts do occur as rare anatomical variants and that they are compatible with normal auditory and vestibular function [20]. It is now clear, however, that such aqueducts can account for oozers but not for gushers.

The widest cochlear aqueduct we have observed in our collection is 0.2 mm in diameter at its narrowest point (fig. 1) which is too small to account for a gusher. Assuming that larger cochlear aqueducts are a possibility, it is doubtful that a gushing flow through the cochlear scalae could occur without tearing Reissner's membrane, an injury that readily occurs during experimental perfusion of animal cochleae (author's experience). Further evidence of the improbability of a gusher passing through the cochlea is that it can occur without causing sensorineural hearing loss. Patent cochlear aqueducts, on the other hand, are logical explanations for oozers. This idea is supported by the fact that oozers (not gushers) are the

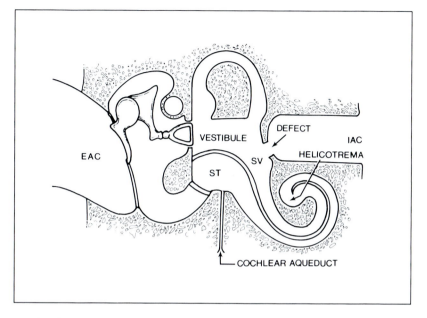

Fig. 2. Diagrammatic sketch showing open fluid pathways from the subarachnoid space to the perilymphatic space. When there is a defect in the fundus of the internal auditory canal, a surgically induced or spontaneous fistula of the oval window will result in a gusher. A patent cochlear aqueduct is too small to accommodate a gusher.

normal result of surgical fenestration of the oval windows of lower mammals (guinea pig, chinchilla, cat) that normally have patent cochlear aqueducts and that the creation of oozers by removing the footplates of these animals does not cause cochlear damage.

The only other logical route for CSF flow into the inner ear is via a bony defect in the fundus of the internal auditory canal. A large amount of fluid could enter the perilymphatic space through such a defect without traversing the cochlear scalae (fig. 2). The first reported histological observation of such a communication occurred in a subject with otopalatodigital syndrome [21] and is listed as case 5 in table I. In an effort to provide further information on the etiology of gushers we have searched our temporal bone collection for evidence of such bony defects. The study included 1,400 temporal bones with fully formed bony labyrinths and 29 with dysmorphic bony labyrinths.

Table I. Dysmorphic bony labyrinths

Case	Age	Ear	Diagnosis	Cochlear aqueduct	Footplates	Modiolus
1	85	R	Mondini	absent	mem defect	
		L	Mondini	absent	mem defect	
2	73	R	Mondini	absent		
		L	Mondini	absent		
3	65	R	Mondini			
		L	Mondini			
4	20	R	Mondini	absent	fixed	
		L	Mondini	absent	absent	
5	2½	R	OPD	absent	fixed	bony defect
6	46 days	R	Klippel-Feil	absent		
		L	Klippel-Feil	absent	fixed	
7	2	R	DiGeorge's	absent		
		L	DiGeorge's	absent		
8	NB	R	DiGeorge's	absent	fixed	
9	NB	L	trisomy 22	absent	absent	
10	NB	R	trisomy 13			
11	10 days	R	trisomy 13–15	absent		
		L	trisomy 13–15	absent		
12	2 weeks	R	trisomy D			
		L	trisomy D			
13	3 months	L	trisomy 13–15		mem defect	
14	3½ months	R	trisomy 18			
		L	trisomy 18			
15	NB	R	anencephaly	absent		
		L	anencephaly	absent	mem defect	bony defect
16	17 days	R	hydantoin	absent	absent	bony defect
		L	hydantoin	absent	fixed	
17	7½ months	R	CHARGE	absent	fixed	
		L	CHARGE	absent	absent	

Fig. 3. Bony defect in the modiolus of a 17-month-old male infant. There is a direct communication from the subarachnoid space of the internal auditory canal and the scala tympani of the basal turn. The defect measures 0.17 mm in vertical diameter.

Fig. 4. Severely dysmorphic labyrinth of a newborn female infant with anencephaly showing a defect of the fundus of the internal auditory canal. It measures 1 × 1 mm in diameter. There is also a membranous area in the footplate of the stapes (fig. 10). Case 15, left ear.

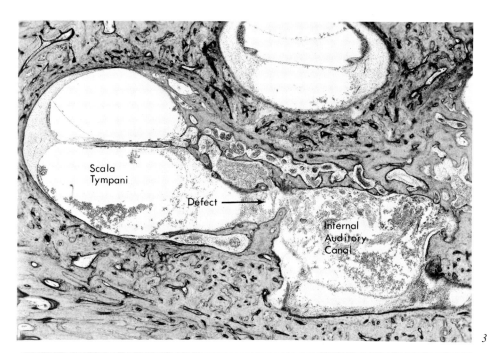

3

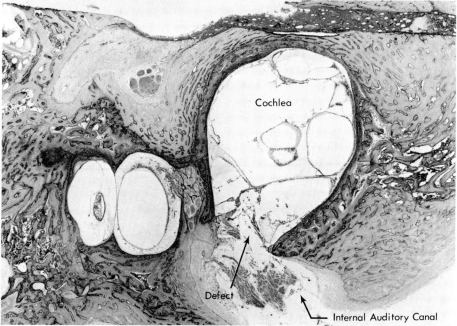

4

Findings

In the group of 1,400 temporal bones having fully formed bony labyrinths only one shows a bony fault in the fundus. It consists of a communication measuring 0.17 mm in vertical diameter (fig. 3) between the internal auditory canal and the scala tympani of the basal turn. It is probably of adequate size to account for an oozer but not a gusher. Failure to find larger defects in fully developed bony labyrinths is not surprising, for the incidence of gushers occurring during stapes surgery appears to be less than 1 per 1,000 (author's experience, 4 in 10,000).

In the collection are 29 temporal bones from 17 subjects showing dysmorphic bony labyrinths (table I). Eighteen of the temporal bones are from subjects having anomalies of other organ systems that were incompatible with prolonged life (cases 7–17). Two temporal bones in this group show modiolar defects resulting in large communications between the internal auditory canals and inner ears. The communicating pathways measure 1 × 1 mm in the left ear of a subject with anencephaly (fig. 4, case 15, left ear) and 2.2 × 2.0 mm in the right ear of a subject with hydantoin syndrome (fig. 5, case 16, right ear). Of the remaining 11 temporal bones from six subjects with normal life expectancies (cases 1–6), an ear from a subject with otopalatodigital syndrome shows a modiolar defect measuring 1.7 × 0.8 mm (fig. 6, case 5, right ear). This ear also has a fixed stapes.

Thus, in the group of 29 temporal bones having dysmorphic bony labyrinths there were three with defects in their modioli of sufficient size to result in a gusher, had the footplate been fenestrated. Only one of these, however, had ossicular pathology and life expectancy that might have eventuated in otologic surgery. Study of the cochlear aqueducts of these 29 temporal bones revealed absent or nonpatent aqueducts in 21. The remaining 8 ears had small (normal-sized) patent aqueducts.

Fig. 5. Markedly deformed labyrinth of a 17-day-old male infant with hydantoin syndrome showing a large defect in the fundus of the internal auditory canal. The defect measures 2.2 × 2.0 mm in diameter. Case 16, right ear.

Fig. 6. Large defect in the fundus of the internal auditory canal and modiolus of a 2½-year-old male child with otopalatodigital syndrome. The channel that leads from the subarachnoid space to the scala vestibuli measures 1.7 × 0.8 mm in diameter. Case 5, right ear.

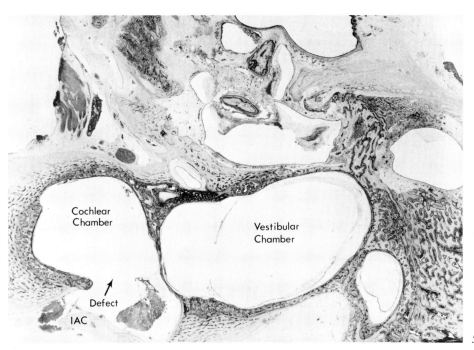

5

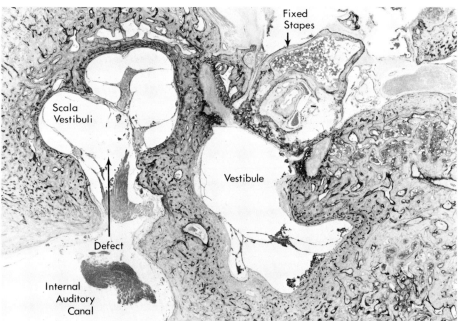

6

Because CSF otorrhea followed by meningitis is a well-recognized complication of the Mondini deformity, we examined the round and oval windows in the 29 dysmorphic ears. The footplates of the stapedes are normal in 15, fixed in 6, absent in 4, and show defects bridged by thin membranes in 4. Two ears with footplate defects are in newborn infants with short life expectancy (trisomy 13–15; anencephaly), and the other two are in both ears of a woman with bilateral Mondini dysplasia who was profoundly deaf from birth and died at the age of 85 (fig. 7–10). In the latter case the fundi of the internal auditory canals have no defects; consequently, the membranes of her faulty footplates were spared the stress of CSF pressure.

Although some of the round window niches contain unresolved mesenchyme, the round window membranes are fully developed in 28 of the 29 ears. In one ear (case 9) the niche is bridged by bone. In no case is there an abnormally large or defective round window membrane.

Surgical Management

Oozers, which we believe are a result of patent cochlear aqueducts, are encountered principally in stapes surgery for otosclerosis. They need not interfere with the completion of surgery and can be controlled without alterations in surgical technique.

Gushers require the application of procedures that will firmly seal the fistulous tracts. Based on clinical experience in dealing with this problem, the senior author (H.F.S.) in a previous publication [22] has recommended the following techniques:

(1) For hearing ears undergoing surgery for conductive hearing loss a two-stage technique can be used. In step 1 the fistula is covered with a fascial graft that is packed in place with a long narrow strip of cloth folded on itself in accordion fashion. The tympanomeatal flap remains elevated and reflected anteriorly. In step 2 (2 or 3 days later) the packing is removed and the tympanomeatal flap is returned to its original position. A prosthe-

---

Fig. 7. Severely dysmorphic labyrinth of an 85-year-old deaf woman. There is a membranous area in the footplate of the stapes. The bracketed area appears at higher magnification in figure 8. Case 1, right ear.

Fig. 8. Bracketed area of figure 7 showing membranous area of the footplate of the stapes. Case 1, right ear.

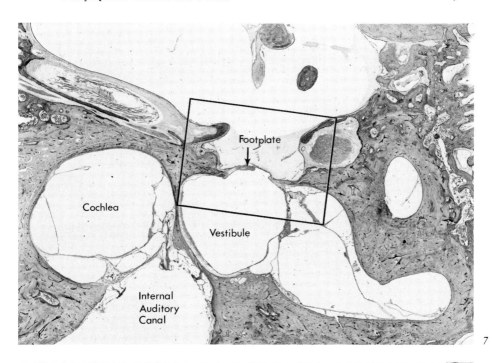

7

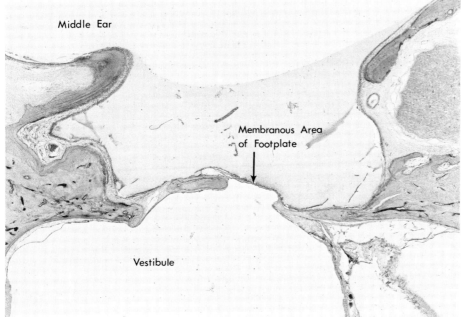

8

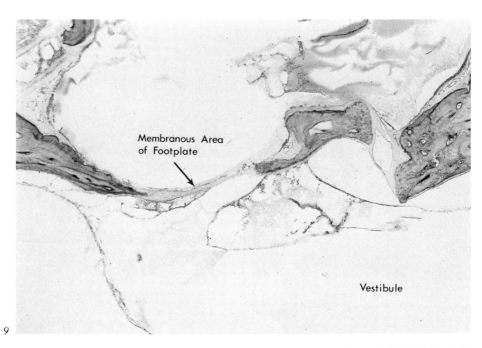

9

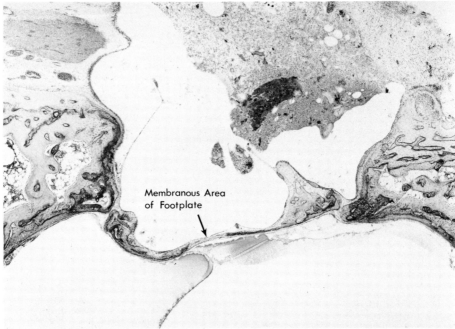

10

sis may be introduced at this time or at a later date. Spontaneous gushers occurring in hearing ears may be treated by the same method.

(2) A simpler one-stage procedure is effective for plugging an oval window fistula for a spontaneous gusher in a nonhearing ear. The defective stapes is removed and the vestibule is packed with subcutaneous fibrous tissue removed from the postauricular area.

Conclusions

Histological study of 1,400 temporal bones with fully developed bony labyrinths and 29 with dysmorphic bony labyrinths support the following conclusions:

(1) The slow welling-type of fluid flow (oozer) that may follow fenestration of the oval window is the result of a wide cochlear aqueduct.

(2) The pouring jet-like outflow (gusher) that may follow fenestration of the oval window is caused by a defect in the fundus of the internal auditory canal that establishes a wide communication between the subarachnoid and perilymphatic spaces.

(3) Fundus defects of sufficient size to cause gushers are rare in fully developed bony labyrinths (none in 1,400 temporal bones in our collection).

(4) Fundus defects of sufficient size to cause gushers occurred in 3 of 29 dysmorphic bony labyrinths (10.3%). For subjects with normal life expectancies and who might have been subjected to surgery for conductive hearing loss had they survived, the incidence was 1 in 11 (0.9%).

(5) Faulty footplate development consisting of partial replacement of the footplate by a thin membrane occurred in 4 of 29 dysmorphic bony labyrinths (13.8%).

(6) When a dysmorphic bony labyrinth has a defect of the fundus of the internal auditory canal as well as a membranous area of the footplate, the constant pressure of cerebrospinal fluid on the membrane can cause distention and rupture of the membrane resulting in spontaneous CSF otorrhea.

Fig. 9. Membranous area in the footplate of the stapes. Case 1, left ear.

Fig. 10. Membranous area in the footplate of the stapes in a newborn female infant with anencephaly. This ear also had a defect in the fundus of the international auditory canal (fig. 4). Case 15, left ear.

References

1 Skolnik, E.M.; Ferrer, J.L.: Cerebrospinal otorrhea. Arch. Otolar. *70:* 795–799 (1959).
2 Rockett, F.X.; Wittenborg, M.H.; Shillito, J., Jr.; Matson, D.D.: Pantopaque visualization of a congenital dural defect of the internal auditory meatus causing rhinorrhea. Report of a case. Am. J. Roentg. *91:* 640–646 (1964).
3 Barr, B.; Wersäll, J.: Cerebrospinal otorrhea with meningitis in congential deafness. Archs Otolar. *81:* 26–28 (1965).
4 Bennett, R.J.: On subarachnoid-tympanic fistulae. A report of two cases of the rare indirect type. J. Laryngol. Otol. *80:* 1242–1252 (1966).
5 Rice, W.J.; Waggoner, L.G.: Congenital cerebrospinal fluid otorrhea via a defect in the stapes footplate. Laryngoscope *77:* 341–349 (1967).
6 Crook, J.P.: Congenital fistula in the stapedial footplate. South. med. J. *60:* 1168–1170 (1967).
7 Kaufman, B.; Jordan, V.M.; Pratt, L.L.: Positive contrast demonstration of a cerebrospinal fluid fistula through the fundus of the internal auditory meatus. Acta radiol. (Diag.) *9:* 83–90 (1969).
8 Gundersen, T.; Haye, R.: Cerebrospinal otorrhea. Archs Otolar. *91:* 19–23 (1970).
9 Schultz, P.; Stool, S.: Recurrent meningitis due to a congenital fistula through the stapes footplate. Am. J. Dis. Child. *120:* 553–554 (1970).
10 Farrior, J.B.; Endicott, J.N.: Congenital mixed deafness. Cerebrospinal fluid otorrhea. Ablation of the aqueduct of the cochlea. Laryngoscope *81:* 684–699 (1971).
11 Stroud, M.H.; Calcaterra, T.C.: Spontaneous perilymph fistulas. Laryngoscope *80:* 479–487 (1970).
12 Nenzelius, C.: On spontaneous cerebrospinal otorrhea due to congenital malformations. Acta oto-lar. *39:* 314–328 (1951).
13 Ward, P.H.: Cerebrospinal fluid otorrhea. Archs Otolar. *74:* 399–404 (1961).
14 Shea, J.J., Jr.: Complications of the stapedectomy operation. Ann. Otol. Rhinol. Lar. *72:* 1109–1123 (1963).
15 Wolferman, S.: Cerebrospinal otorrhea, a complication of stapes surgery. Laryngoscope *74:* 1368–1380 (1964).
16 Sooy, F.A.: The management of middle ear lesions simulating otosclerosis. Ann. Otol. Rhinol. Lar. *69:* 540–558 (1960).
17 Olson, N.R.; Lehman, R.H.: Cerebrospinal fluid otorrhea and the congenitally fixed stapes. Laryngoscope *78:* 352–360 (1968).
18 Buran, D.J.; Duvall, A.J., III: The oto-palato-digital (OPD) syndrome. Archs Otolar. *85:* 394–399 (1967).
19 Glasscock, M.E.; III: The stapes gusher. Archs Otolar. *98:* 82–91 (1973).
20 Schuknecht, H.F.: Pathology of the ear (Harvard University Press, Cambridge 1974).
21 Shi, S.-R.: Temporal bone findings in a case of otopalatodigital syndrome. Archs Otolar. *111:* 119–121 (1985).
22 Schuknecht, H.F.: Mondini dysplasia. A clinical and pathological study. Ann. Otol. Rhinol. Lar. *89:* suppl. 65, pp. 1–23 (1980).

Harold F. Schuknecht, MD, Department of Otolaryngology,
Massachusetts Eye and Ear Infirmary, 243 Charles Street, Boston, MA 02114 (USA)

Adv. Oto-Rhino-Laryng., vol. 39, pp. 13–17 (Karger, Basel 1988)

Improvements of a Method for Testing Autoantibodies in Sensorineural Hearing Loss[1]

A.M. Soliman, F. Zanetti

Department of Otorhinolaryngology, University of Tübingen, Tübingen, FRG

Introduction

Humoral antibodies against various cellular components were demonstrated in serum of patients with immune-mediated vestibulo-cochlear disorders [2, 5, 7]. The immunofluorescence test (IF) applied for detecting these autoantibodies utilized frozen preparations from human kidney and thyroid, as well as frozen sections of mouse kidney, liver, stomach and heart muscles [2, 5]. Frozen preparations are considered optimal for immunofluorescent optical examination [8]. Elies and Plester (1983, 1985) first reported the use of cochlear tissue from young hamsters and rats, together with other tissues, as antigenic substrates in the IF [1, 2]. The frozen cochlear tissue, however, is difficult to section due to the nondecalcified bony elements. Moreover, floating and dispersion of the frozen sections during the different phases of incubation is not uncommon [6, 9]. It was reported that in addition to the bright fluorescence of the nondecalcified cochlear bone, the basilar membrane, the stria vascularis and even the organ of Corti reveal a strong autofluorescence in frozen sections of hamster's cochlea. The weak immunological reaction with patients' sera and the unclear cochlear morphology led to the conclusion that frozen kidney preparations are more sensitive and reliable for testing such autoantibodies.

The aim of this study is to present the results of applying antibody-positive and negative human serum controls, as well as sera from patients with sensorineural hearing loss (SNHL) to the IF, using frozen nondecalcified cochlear preparations from young hamsters as the antigenic sub-

[1] Supported by Deutsche Forschungsgemeinschaft, grant PL 79/5.

strate. A number of modifications are described and the significance of some new interesting findings are discussed in the light of the presented modifications.

Materials and Methods

Young golden hamsters (14 days old, 50–100 g) were deeply anesthetized with intra-peritoneal Nembutal® (3 mg/100 g body weight). Both cochleas were intravitally frozen by immersing the head in liquid nitrogen. The animal was immediately decapitated and the frozen head was sectioned and trimmed with an electric-saw so that only the middle third of the head enclosing the temporal bone remained. The trimmed head was mounted to a WK 1150 cryotome and sectioned until the cochlea was identified. The tissue around the mounted cochlea was carefully trimmed using a small handsaw so that the frozen cochlea was surrounded only by a thin rim of soft tissue. Sectioning was then done at $-20\,°C$ without difficulty. The 10-μm sections were fixed with $4\,°C$ cold acetone. The sections were ready for use in the IF.

The IF was done according to the method of Mackay and Ritts [4]. The frozen cochlear sections were incubated with: (1) Negative human sera for the detection of non-specific fluorescence. (2) Antibody-positive human sera with antibodies against mito-chondria, nuclei and nucleoli (Kallstad, Freiburg). These sera were used as markers for testing the immunological reactivity of the applied cochlear tissue. (3) Sera from 5 patients with SNHL.

The incubation was done at room temperature followed by wash in phosphate-buffered saline (PBS, pH 7.4). Sections were then covered with a 1:36 dilution of fluores-cein-labelled antihuman immunoglobulins developed in sheep (Wellcome Diagnostics). After appropriate wash in PBS, the sections were mounted in buffered polyvinyl alcohol (PVA, Kallstad, Freiburg) and examined under a Zeiss fluorescence microscope.

Results

Incubation of frozen nondecalcified sections of young golden hamsters' cochlea with antibody-positive human serum models demonstrated a strong specific fluorescence, always corresponding to the serum model applied. The fine granular fluorescence of the mitochondria, the bright dot-like nucleolar reaction and the homogenous nuclear fluorescence were clearly revealed against a dark background (fig. 1a–c). A positive reaction was present all over the cochlea and within the cells of the various cochlear structures: the limbus spiralis, the stria vascularis, the spiral ligament, the spiral ganglion, the modiolar vessels and the organ of Corti. Even some vestibular structures which could be obtained in the frozen sections revealed a similar specific reaction (fig. 2a, b).

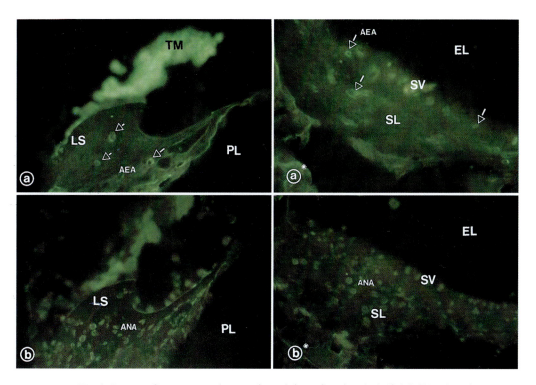

Fig. 4. Immunofluorescent microscopic staining of anti-endothelial (AEA, *a*) and (ANA, *b*) antibodies in serum of patients with SNHL. The AEA reaction appears as bright fluorescence of the capillary endothelium in the limbus spiralis *(a)* and the stria vascularis *(a*)*. The ANA reaction revealed in the limbus spiralis *(b)*, stria vascularis and the spiral ligament *(b*)* is of the homogeneous form. ✕ 31.

On the other hand, when the IF was carried out using normal human sera as a control, the structures mentioned above appeared dark and showed no fluorescence. The tectorial membrane and the nondecalcified cochlear bone were the only structures revealing a constant nonspecific fluorescence (fig. 3a, b).

Applying sera from 5 patients with SNHL revealed anti-endothelial antibodies (AEA) in one serum and a weak antinuclear reaction (ANA) in another. The remaining 3 sera were negative to antibodies matching the negative serum control. The AEA were seen as a bright fluorescence of the vascular endothelium in both the strial capillaries and the modiolar vessels. Similar vascular fluorescence could be detected in the limbus spiralis, the spiral ligament and occasionally in the spiral ganglion (fig. 4a, a*). We found no difficulty in spotting the weak nuclear reaction, which appeared as a homogeneous fluorescence, in the serum of a patient under cortisone therapy (fig. 4b, b*). The cochlear architecture was well preserved in the nondecalcified preparations and the structural details of the different cochlear elements were clearly delineated.

Discussion

In this report a number of modifications were applied aiming at improving the quality of the cochlear sections, preventing the floating and dispersion during incubation and improving the immunological reliability of the frozen cochlear tissue in detecting autoantibodies in patients with inner ear disorders. The modifications could be summarized in three points: (1) Meticulous trimming of the mounted frozen cochlea at $-20\,°C$. (2) Fixation of the sections in a $4\,°C$ cold acetone instead of 4% gelatin. (3) Mounting of the incubated nondecalcified preparations in PVA instead of the conventional PBS-glycerine.

The ossification of the temporal bone of golden hamsters, in contrast to other experimental animals, is not complete up to the 16th day after birth. By this time the bony cochlea is soft and thin [3]. This, combined with the complete trimming of the surrounding bone and tissue made it possible to section the nondecalcified cochlea without much difficulty. The cochlear architecture was also preserved.

Fixation of the frozen sections in cold acetone proved to be superior to embedding them in 4% gelatin. A darker background was always obtained. The color contrast between the bright fluorescence and a dark background enabled the detection of even a weak positive reaction. Moreover, the cold acetone fixation aided in minimizing the floating of cochlear sections during incubation.

Substituting the PBS-glycerine with PVA as a mounting medium proved to be advantageous in avoiding the dispersion and destruction of the incubated preparations before microscopic examination. We do believe that this advantage offered by PVA is merely due to its physical properties and not to the difference in chemical composition.

In contrast to previous reports applying the same type of frozen cochlear tissue, the basilar membrane, the stria vascularis and the spiral ligament revealed no nonspecific fluorescence in our preparations. These structures reacted specifically with the different antibodies as demonstrated by incubation with the antibody-positive serum models and the patients' sera. Embedding the cochlear sections in gelatin alone or dryness of the frozen preparations might explain these previous findings.

An interesting finding was the false fluorescence sometimes revealed by the neural modiolar structures and by the brain tissue. Neural elements and brain tissue should therefore be used with care for evaluation of the IF results. It should be taken into consideration that the detected antibodies are not organ-specific, and that they could be detected by using other forms of tissues.

In summary, frozen nondecalcified cochlear preparations from young gold hamsters proved to be as sensitive as other tissues (e.g. kidney) in detecting humoral antibodies in serum of patients with SNHL. Moreover, they offer the advantage of testing the debatable existence of inner ear specific antibodies simultaneously. They are reliable when used as antigenic substrates in the IF. Trimming of the mounted frozen cochlea, fixation in acetone and gelatin and mounting in PVA proved to be advantageous in improving the quality of the frozen sections, minimizing the floating of sections during incubation, delineating the fine cochlear structural details and revealing the immunological reliability of the applied cochlear tissue.

References

1   Elies, W.: Immunologische Befunde bei cochleo-vestibulären Störungen. Allergologie *6:* 357–361 (1983).
2   Elies, W.; Plester, D.: In Veldman, McCabe, Huizing, Mygind, Immunobiology, autoimmunity and transplantation in otorhinolaryngology, pp. 111–117 (Kugler, Amsterdam 1985).

3   Giebel, W.: Chemische Analysen der Innenohrflüssigkeiten und histochemische Enzymnachweise an Innenohrgeweben von Säugetieren und einzelnen niederen Vertebraten sowie Untersuchungen der Eigenbewegung der Innenohrflüssigkeit des Meerschweinchens; Habschr., Tübingen (1981).

4   Mackay, I.R.; Ritts, R.E.: WHO handbook of immunological techniques, vol. 9, p. II (World Health Organisation, Geneva 1979).

5   Plester, D.; Zanetti, F.; Berg, P.A.; Klein, R.: Diagnostic laboratory tools for immune-mediated sensorineural hearing loss. Proc. 2nd Int. Academic Conf. in Immunobiology, Utrecht, in press.

6   Soliman, A.M.: An improved technique for the study of immunofluorescence using nondecalcified guinea pig cochlea. J. Lar. Otol. (in press).

7   Soliman, A.M.: The use of immunofluorescence in the non-decalcified frozen guinea pig cochlea to detect autoantibodies in inner ear disorders. Archs Oto-Rhino-Lar. *244:* 241–245 (1987).

8   Thoenes, G.H.: Die Immunhistologie der Glomerulonephritis. Klin. Wschr. *51:* 739–747 (1973).

9   Wei, N.R.; Giebel, W.; Plester, D.; Schrader, M.: Zur Verwendung von Cochleagewebe von Goldhamster und Mensch zur Auswertung humoraler Antikörper bei Innenohrerkrankungen. Archs Oto-Rhino-Lar., suppl. II, pp. 165–167 (1986).

Dr. A.M. Soliman, Hals-Nasen-Ohrenklinik der Universität Tübingen, Silcherstrasse 5, D–7400 Tübingen (FRG)

Adv. Oto-Rhino-Laryng., vol. 39, pp. 18–36 (Karger, Basel 1988)

The Eustachian Tube Profile in Children

A Quantitative Histopathological Study of the ET Lumen and
Mucosal Lining Involvement in Acute and Secretory Otitis Media[1]

J. Sadé, M. Luntz, G. Berger

Department of Otolaryngology, Meir Hospital, Kfar Saba, Sackler School of
Medicine, Tel Aviv University, Tel Aviv, Israel

Introduction

Acute and secretory otitis media (AOM and SOM) are often considered to be secondary to inflammatory obstruction or narrowing of the eustachian tube (ET), leading to inadequate middle ear aeration [1–5]. However, no one has yet demonstrated anatomical obstruction of the ET in
humans, or presented quantitative data based on measurements of the ET
lumen, that would indicate a significant tubal narrowing in inflamed ears.
Thus, in order to obtain such conclusive evidence of the ET lumen involvement, a systematic measurement of the ET lumen size of normal and
inflamed temporal bones and a comparison between the two groups has
been made [6–12].

The ET is a complicated and irregular organ, changing its size and
inner contour along its course, a feature posing a methodological problem
when measuring the lumen. To solve this problem we have arbitrarily

[1] This paper is a synthesis of several experimental studies carried out in the last 5
years. The investigations were undertaken in collaboration with: Dr. A. Shabtai, Dr. S.
Wolfson, Dr. Z. Sachs, Dr. I. Levit and especially Mrs. M. Haimovich, Mrs. D. Lerman
and Miss I. Garlenter.

divided the ET into six different anatomical segments (pharyngeal, mid-portion, near-isthmus, isthmus, post-isthmus and pre-tympanum). Each one has its own characteristics as to the shape of the lumen as well as to other specific enveloping features [13]. The division of the ET into six segments provided constant points of reference and enabled us to compare the cross-sectional areas of corresponding regions of normal ears with those of ears retrieved from temporal bones with acute and secretory otitis media.

We took the view that a thorough investigation of the ET involvement in otitis media must also encompass an assessment of the histopathological changes affecting its walls. This includes quantitative data on the distribution and the extent of the inflammatory reaction along the tubal walls in each of its six segments. Moreover, we decided to extend the study of the mucosal inflammatory changes to the middle ear, in order to compare the magnitude of inflammation between the two organs.

Material and Methods

Lumen Size Measurements

Sixty-one temporal bones (TBs) – 17 of the bones included the entire length of the ET, while 44 contained only certain segments of the ET – were processed for histological studies. They were removed from patients whose ages ranged from newborn to 2 years. Forty-two of the bones did not exhibit any middle ear pathology and were therefore considered as normal. Of the remaining 19 TBs, 13 showed histological changes compatible with AOM and 6 with SOM.

The TBs were fixed in formalin and decalcified with 3% nitric acid. Once decalcification became advanced, each TB was trimmed and cut into four blocks that were further decalcified. Following decalcification, the blocks were rinsed with water and immersed in 20% sodium sulfate solution to neutralize and remove excessive acid. Dehydration was carried out with increasing concentrations of ethanol, and thereafter the blocks were embedded in paraffin and serially sectioned. Ten-micrometer thick sections were stained with hematoxylin-eosin, periodic acid-Sciff and Masson's trichrome.

As described previously, the ET was divided into six segments to ensure an accurate comparison between similar regions. The following section depicts the characteristics of each one of these segments.

(1) The Pharyngeal Portion (fig. 1, 2). The pharyngeal portion is the most antero-medial segment of the ET. There it opens into the nasopharynx, while postero-laterally it blends with the midportion of the tube. It is a relatively long segment, ranging from 4 mm in infants to 9 mm in adults. The shape of its lumenal cross-section in a cadaver has a slit-like appearance, and it is curved in a semi-lunar fashion. The epithelial lining is respiratory in type. It is surrounded by abundant glands medially and laterally.

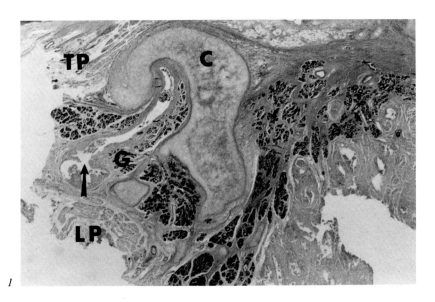

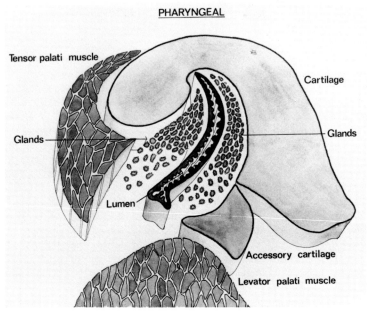

Fig. 1. A cross-section through the pharyngeal portion. Arrow = Lumen; C = cartilage; G = glands; TP = tensor palati muscle; LP = levator palati muscle, PAS. × 10.5.
Fig. 2. A schematic drawing of a cross-section through the pharyngeal portion.

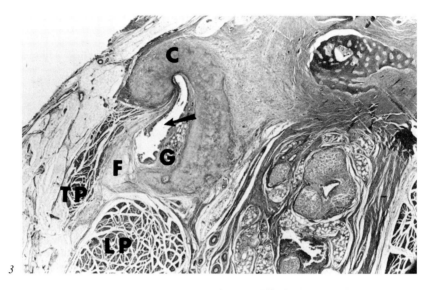

3

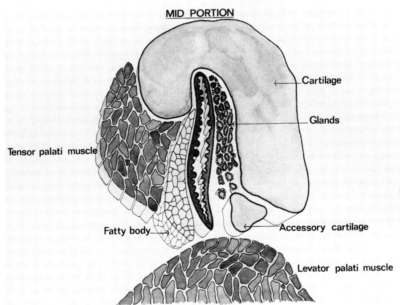

4

Fig. 3. A cross-section through the mid-portion. Arrow = Lumen; C = cartilage; G = glands; F = fatty body; TP = tensor palati muscle; LP = levator palati muscle. PAS. × 10.5.

Fig. 4. A schematic drawing through the mid-portion.

The tube framework is cartilaginous both medially and superiorily, while its inferior and lateral aspects are bordered by the levator palati muscle and the tensor palati muscle, respectively. Often, small accessory cartilaginous parts are seen at the lower end.

(2) The Midportion (fig. 3, 4). The midportion comes next to the pharyngeal portion. Its length ranges from 4 mm in infants to 8 mm in adults. Its lumenal cross-section in the cadaver is similarly slit-like and curved. The epithelium is also respiratory in type, especially along the floor. In the subepithelial connective tissue, glands are seen only medially, laterally they are replaced by an impressive fatty tissue. The outer cartilaginous framework now has the classical shepherd's crook form, extending from the top of the tube to cover its medial aspect. Both the levator and the tensor palati muscles are well developed.

(3) The Near-Isthmus (fig. 5, 6). The near-isthmus is the third part of the ET. It was already recognized by Zollner [15] as a specific segment and was termed 'the physiological isthmus'. It is a short segment, ranging from 2 mm in infants to 4 mm in adults. Its lumenal cross-section is no more slit-like and curved, but almond-shaped. The epithelium is respiratory in type and the medially situated subepithelial connective tissue has become very thin and devoid of glands. The lateral fatty tissue is gradually being replaced by fibrous tissue. Cartilaginous tissue is still found to border the subepithelial connective tissue superiorily and medially, though the medial vertical plate is considerably shortened. In fact, the more one goes posteriorily, the more one finds the cartilage to be gradually replaced by the petrous temporal bone. While inferiorily the levator palati is seen to be very prominent, the laterally situated tensor palati muscle is almost completely replaced by its tendon. The internal carotid artery is always found about 5 mm medial to the near-isthmus lumen.

(4) The Isthmus (fig. 7, 8). While the first three segments account for about two-thirds of the tubal length and constitute the part which is dilated by the tubal muscles, the isthmus is the beginning of the rigid part as well as the narrowest of all segments. This narrow zone, i.e. the isthmus, is not a point where cartilage stops and the bony part begins, but extends for about 2 mm in the infant and 4 mm in the adult. Its lumenal cross-section has an oval configuration; however, there is a marked inconsistency in the isthmic lumen shape, and only a few specimens disclose a perfectly oval form. The epithelial lining is respiratory in type. The thin subepithelial connective tissue is bounded superiorily by a cap of cartilage, and the rest of its circumference is surrounded by the petrous temporal bone. The tensor and the levator palati muscles have disappeared completely. The tensor tympani muscle makes its appearance above the isthmic lumen, yet plenty of bone or cartilage interpose between it and the lumen. The internal carotid artery is seen about 1.5 mm medial to the isthmic lumen.

(5) The Post-Isthmus (fig. 9, 10). The post-isthmus constitutes the fifth segment of the ET. Antero-medially it blends with the isthmus and postero-laterally it communicates with the pre-tympanic portion of the tube. This is also a short segment, ranging from 1.5 mm in infants to 3.5 mm in adults. The lumen's triangular-like cross-sectional shape differs from both the oval shape of the isthmus and the rectangular-like appearance of the next successive segment, the pre-tympanum. The epithelial lining is respiratory in type. The thin subepithelial connective tissue is surrounded by the petrous temporal bone; however, especially in infants, some cartilage is often present as a small cap along the roof. The tensor tympani muscle is seen superiorily, separated from the lumen by the cartilage. The internal carotid artery lies medio-inferior to the lumen, about 1.5 mm from it.

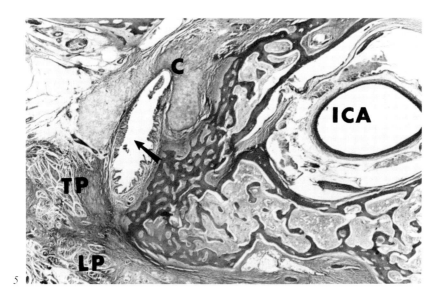

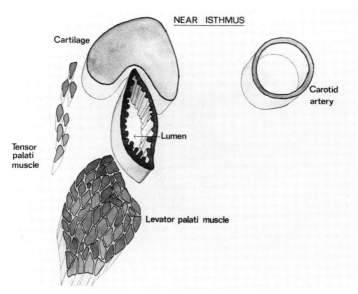

Fig. 5. A cross-section through the near-isthmus. Arrow = Lumen; C = cartilage; TP = tensor palati muscle; LP = levator palati muscle; ICA = internal carotid artery. PAS. × 10.5.

Fig. 6. A schematic drawing of a cross-section through the near-isthmus.

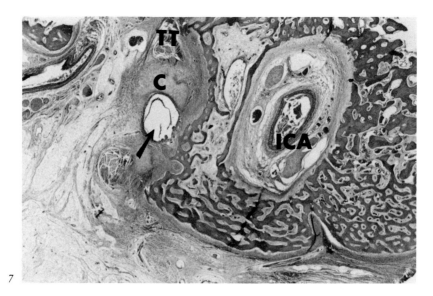

7

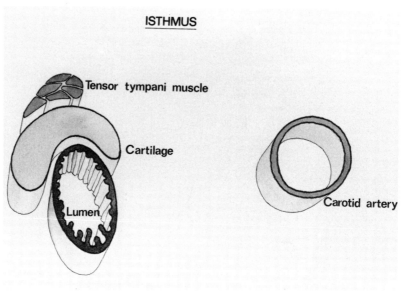

8

Fig. 7. A cross-section through the isthmus. Arrow = Lumen; C = cartilage; TT = tensor tympani muscle; ICA = internal carotid artery. PAS. × 10.5.

Fig. 8. A schematic drawing of a cross-section through the isthmus.

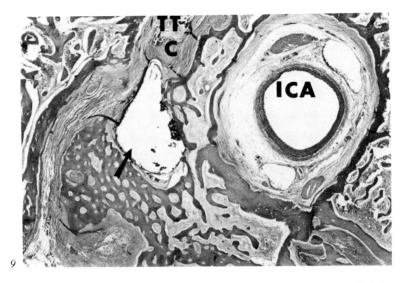

9

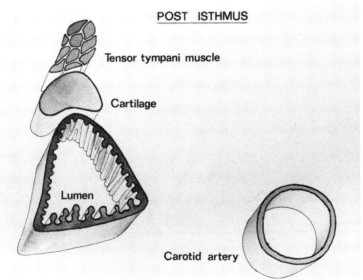

10

Fig. 9. A cross-section through the post-isthmus. Arrow = Lumen; C = cartilage; TT = tensor tympani muscle; ICA = internal carotid artery. PAS. × 10.5.

Fig. 10. A schematic drawing of a cross-section through the post-isthmus.

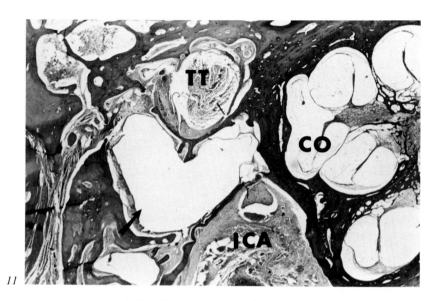

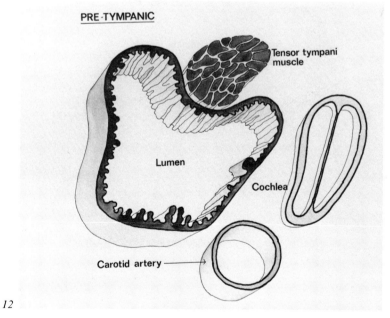

Fig. 11. A cross-section through the pre-tympanic area. Arrow = Lumen; TT = tensor tympani muscle; ICA = internal carotid artery; Co = cochlea. PAS. × 10.5.

Fig. 12. A schematic drawing of a cross-section through the pre-tympanic region.

(6) The Pre-Tympanum (fig. 11, 12). The pre-tympanic segment is the most postero-lateral part of the ET, blending antero-medially with the post-isthmus and opening into the tympanum. It is a relatively long segment, ranging from 4 mm in infants to 9 mm in adults. Its lumenal cross-section has a rectangular-like shape. It is covered by a respiratory type of epithelium. The thin subepithelial connective tissue is surrounded by the petrous temporal bone; however, a small remnant of cartilage may at times continue along the roof all the way up to the middle ear. This cartilaginous cap is present mainly in children, but can occasionally also be found in adults. Supero-medially the tensor tympani muscle is separated from the lumen by a thin plate of bone. The muscle is so well developed in this part, that it bulges supero-medially into the lumen, creating the typical convex shaped roof of the pre-tympanic lumen. The medial wall of the pretympanic region bears constant relationship with both the internal carotid artery and the anterior 'tip' of the cochlea. The internal carotid artery is found infero-medially to the more antero-medial part of the pre-tympanum, separated from the lumen by a very thin plate of bone less than 1 mm in width. Occasionally, no bone but fibrous tissue separates the artery and the lumen of the pre-tympanum. The anterior part of the cochlear basal coil is found medial to the most postero-lateral portion of the pre-tympanic segment.

Measurements of the lumenal cross-sectional area of each one of the six segments were carried out with the aid of a light microscope fitted with a viewer on which a special grid was mounted. This set up enabled precise measurements down to one hundredth of a millimeter (fig. 13, 14).

The Student's t test was applied to compare the lumen areas of normal and pathological temporal bones.

Assessment of the Tubal Wall Involvement in Otitis media

Thirty-seven TBs were included in the study. Seventeen bones from infants aged 1 day to 18 months (mean age 6 months), disclosed inflammatory involvement of the middle ear cleft. Of the 17 pathological bones, 13 demonstrated changes compatible with acute and 4 with secretory otitis media. The remaining 20 TBs, from patients aged 6 months to 10 years (mean age 3 years), did not exhibit any middle ear pathology and served as normal controls.

The TBs underwent the same processing as described before. Representative sections from the middle ear and from each one of the 6 segments of the ET were studied. Two parameters of the tubal and the middle ear inflammatory response were estimated: (1) the proportion of the circumference involved by inflammation, and (2) the inflammatory swelling of the mucosal lining.

A preliminary study revealed that the edema and the inflammatory cell infiltration which characterize the inflammatory response of the middle ear and the ET are confined to the subepithelial connective tissue. This connective tissue lies adjacent to the epithelium, while glands as well as fatty tissue are located more peripherally. Since the inflammatory response did not extend beyond this layer of connective tissue, it was thought that a comparison between the thickness of this layer in normal and pathological specimens would provide a quantitative insight as to the extent of the inflammatory swelling in the middle ear and at various sites of the ET. In order to achieve standardization of the tubal measurements, two problems had to be tackled. First, the inner border of the connective tissue layer within which the inflammatory reaction took place had to be accurately identified. It was outlined by a dense layer of fibrous tissue, clearly visible with haematoxylin-

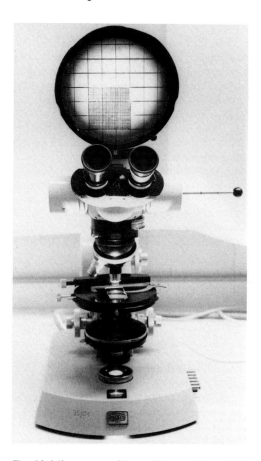

Fig. 13. Microscope with a grid mounted on its top.

eosin and PAS stains. The second problem was the marked irregularity of the tubal wall's inflammatory involvement which made any attempt to find a mean value of the tubal wall thickness impossible. This problem was solved by calculating the mean value of the tubal wall thickness at four constant points: the upper and lower poles, and the middle of the medial and lateral walls (fig. 15). These problems did not exist in the middle ear where the border of the connective tissue layer is the easily identified periosteum, and the inflammatory reaction is distributed rather evenly throughout most of the circumference.

The aforementioned considerations allowed quantification and comparison between the inflammatory involvement of the middle ear and the six segments of the ET.

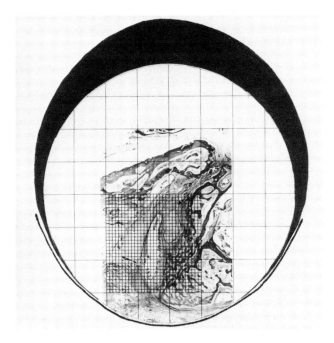

Fig. 14. A microscopic section of the ET (mid-portion) under the grid. Note: each mini square represents one hundredth square millimeter.

Results

Lumen Size Measurements

Examination of all the TBs with AOM and SOM revealed that the patency of the lumen was maintained throughout the entire length of the ET. This excludes the possibility that middle ear inflammation is associated with an organic obstruction of the ET [6–12].

The measurements of the lumenal cross-sectional area of these segments indicate that: (1) there is a considerable variation of lumen size within each age group in the normal as well as in the pathological TBs; (2) in all the six segments the mean lumen size of normal specimens was found to be larger than that of the pathological ones (table I). However, this difference was found to be statistically insignificant.

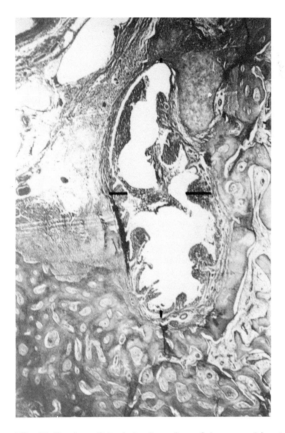

Fig. 15. Section of the isthmic region of the eustachian tube. The mean thickness of the mucosal lining of the upper and lower poles and at the middle of the medial and lateral walls (black bars) was used for comparison between normal and inflamed specimens. PAS. × 70.

Assessment of the Tubal Wall Involvement in Otitis media

The submucosa of the ET and middle ear of TB with AOM and SOM displays edema of the subepithelial connective tissue with numerous engorged and dilated blood vessels. The edematous connective tissue is diffusely infiltrated with polymorphonuclear leucocytes in acute otitis media, and with mononuclear cells (macrophages, lymphocytes and plasma cells) in secretory otitis media. Other occasional features of tubal and middle ear inflammation include increased subepithelial glandular

Table I. Cross-sectional area of ET lumina (mean ± SD)

Segment	Luminal cross-sectional area, mm^2		p
	normal specimens	pathological specimens	
Pharyngeal	0.72 ± 0.43 (n = 29)	0.70 ± 0.46 (n = 14)	0.912
Midportion	0.66 ± 0.35 (n = 37)	0.64 ± 0.39 (n = 15)	0.889
Near-isthmus	0.60 ± 0.41 (n = 31)	0.49 ± 0.33 (n = 17)	0.349
Isthmus	1.06 ± 0.78 (n = 36)	0.73 ± 0.37 (n = 15)	0.124
Post-isthmus	2.19 ± 1.42 (n = 29)	1.57 ± 0.80 (n = 15)	0.123
Pre-tympanum	5.33 ± 1.97 (n = 28)	4.48 ± 1.94 (n = 13)	0.205

Table II. Proportion of the tubal and middle ear circumference involved with inflammation

Region	% involvement
Pharyngeal	42
Midportion	40
Near-isthmus	51
Isthmus	51
Post-isthmus	52
Pre-tympanum	62
Middle ear	93

formation and conspicuous intraluminal projections of folds or villi consisting of reactive epithelium and subepithelial connective tissue.

The distribution of the inflammatory response of the ET in acute as well as in secretory otitis media is characterized by a marked irregularity. At any given segment of the tube the inflammatory reaction is not homogeneous but shows a rather irregular pattern *usually involving only a portion of the circumference.* In contrast to the ET, the middle ear exhibits a more homogeneous pattern of involvement, wherein the mucosal inflammatory response is almost the same everywhere. The proportion of the tubal and the middle ear circumference involved with inflammation is shown in table II. The tubal involvement ranges between 40% of the midportion and 62% of the pre-tympanic portion, whereas the middle ear is involved almost throughout its circumference (93%).

The measurements of the subepithelial connective tissue reveal that the pathological specimens are thicker than the normal; the difference between them represents the inflammatory swelling. Moreover, we calculated the ratio between the inflammatory swelling and the thickness of the normal specimen to demonstrate the relative increase in the thickness of the inflamed specimen. Table III shows the relative increase in the thickness of the middle ear and the six segments of the ET. It is evident that the maximal increase in the thickness of the subepithelial connective tissue occurs in the middle ear, whereas the ET is involved to a lesser extent. Within the latter there is a marked difference between the bony segments (isthmus, post-isthmus, and pre-tympanum) and the cartilaginous ones (pharyngeal, midportion and near-isthmus). The inflammatory involvement of the former exceeds that of the latter. Figure 16 demonstrates the gradual decrease in the magnitude of the inflammatory reaction from the middle ear towards the pharyngeal orifice of the tube.

Table III. Increase in the mean mucosal thickness of 17 inflamed specimens

Region	% increase in mucosal thickness
Pharyngeal	78
Midportion	38
Near-isthmus	50
Isthmus	91
Post-isthmus	133
Pre-tympanum	259
Middle ear	400

Fig. 16. Temporal bone of an infant with acute otitis media. a Section of the middle ear promontory. There is an extensive edema and inflammatory cell infiltration of the subepithelial connective tissue. BW = Bony wall of the promontory, ME = middle ear space, PAS. × 70. b Section of the post-isthmic region representing the bony segments of the tube. The inflammatory response occupies the inferior wall and is less pronounced than that of the middle ear. BW = Bony wall of the tube, C = cartilage at the tubal roof; L = tubal lumen. PAS. × 70. c Section of the near-isthmic region representing the cartilaginous segments of the tube. The inflammatory response is minimal. C = Tubal cartilage; arrow = tubal lumen. PAS. × 70.

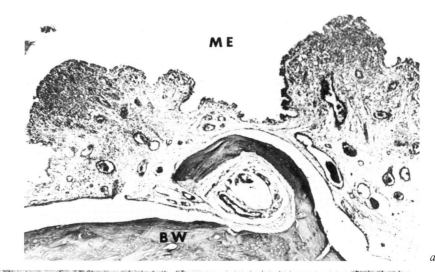

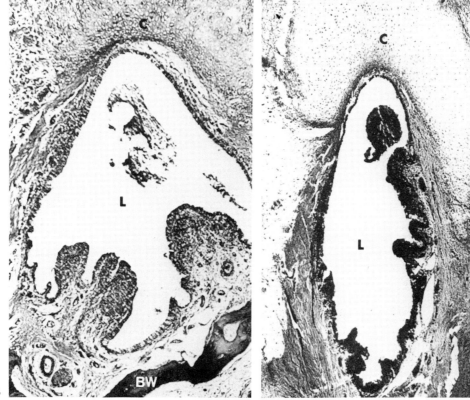

Discussion

The pathogenesis of AOM and SOM has frequently been attributed to obstruction or narrowing of the ET. The blocked tube causes inadequate aeration, an ex vacuo phenomenon, leading to accumulation of an effusion within the tympanic cavity, and defective clearance of the middle ear. However, no one has yet demonstrated anatomical obstruction of the auditory tube in humans. In fact, there are studies that negate the obstruction hypothesis. Thus, Sadé [16] did not find ET obstruction in a histological study of TBs removed from patients with SOM. Moreover, when Sadé et al. [17] inserted ventilating tubes into the eardrums of patients with SOM, they observed that the middle ears cleared in a few days without external drainage of the effusion. This would indicate that the ET remained open and allowed the effusion to drain through it once a 'counter opening' was performed.

Although our study establishes that in AOM and SOM the ET is not obstructed, the probability that its lumen is narrowed down is still a possible explanation for the aeration deficiency. The present study shows that histologically, the ET is patent throughout its length in AOM and SOM and there is no statistically significant difference between normal and inflamed specimens – as far as the size of their ET lumen. However, from table I one can see that a consistent trend exists disclosing narrowing of the ET lumen of the inflamed TBs when compared to the normal TBs. This difference increases monotonically (in absolute values) from the pharyngeal portion to the pretympanic region. In the first three segments the difference is very small – while in the last three (those which are closer to the middle ear) it becomes more pronounced (table I). It should be pointed out that had our material consisted of a larger number of TBs, the difference between the two lumens' size of the healthy and inflamed TBs might have been found to be statistically significant. It is indeed our intention to enlarge the number of the studied TBs with the view of establishing this point.

The measurements of the subepithelial connective tissue in specimens with AOM and SOM clearly indicate that a significant dissimilarity exists between the tubal and the middle ear inflammatory reaction. While the ET inflammation is characterized by a patchy, haphazard and irregular distribution, that of the middle ear is more homogeneous. Moreover, the magnitude of the middle ear inflammatory involvement at any given spot is considerably greater (several orders of magnitude!) than that of the tube. Thus, the modest involvement of the ET implies that the tube plays a role of only a minor partner in otitis media. These findings are supported by the work of Kitajiri et al. [18] who reported that the severity of the middle ear inflammation is greater than that of the tube in patients with cleft and high arched palates. On the other hand, they differ from Zechner's comment that the morphological changes in both sites are very similar [19].

From the above it is evident that both in AOM as in SOM the ET plays some part in the middle ear inflammation, yet it probably plays only a 'second fiddle' in the pathogenesis of acute and secretory otitis media.

References

1 Bluestone, C.D.; Casselbrant, M.L.; Cantekin, E.I.: Functional obstruction of the eustachian tube in the pathogenesis of aural cholesteatoma in children; in Sadé, Cholesteatoma and mastoid surgery, pp. 211–224 (Kugler, Amsterdam 1982).

2 Holmquist, J.; Renvall, U.: Eustachian tube function in secretory otitis media. Archs Otolar. 99: 59–61 (1974).

3 Sadé, J.: Eustachian tube function; in Sadé, Secretory otitis media and its sequelae, pp. 212–253 (Churchill Livingstone, New York 1979).

4 Tos, M.; Wiederhold, M.; Larsen, P.: Experimental long term tubal occlusion in cats. Acta oto-lar. 97: 580–592 (1984).

5 Beery, Q.C.; Doyle, W.J.; Cantekin, E.I.; Bluestone, C.D.: Longitudinal assessment of eustachian tube function in children. Laryngoscope 89: 1446–1456 (1979).

6 Sadé, J.; Wolfson, S.; Galrenter, I.; Luntz, M.: The eustachian tube lumen in acute and secretory otitis media; in Sadé, The eustachian tube, pp. 41–48 (Kugler, Amsterdam 1987).

7 Sadé, J.; Wolfson, S.; Sachs, Z.; Levit, I.; Abraham, S.: The infant's eustachian tube lumen: the pharyngeal part. J. Lar. Otol. 100: 129–134 (1986).

8 Sadé, J.; Wolfson, S.; Sachs, Z.; Abraham, S.: The eustachian tube midportion in infants. Am. J. Otolaryngol. 6: 205–209 (1985).

9 Sadé, J.; Wolfson, S.; Sachs, Z.; Abraham, S.: Caliber of the lumen of the eustachian tube pre-isthmus in infants and children. Archs Otolar. 242: 247–255 (1985).

10 Sadé, J.; Wolfson, S.; Sachs, Z.; Levit, I.; Abraham, S.: The human eustachian tube lumen in children. I. The isthmus. Acta oto-lar. 99: 305–309 (1985).

11 Sadé, J.; Luntz, M.; Berger, G.: The infant's 'post-isthmus' region of the eustachian tube in health and disease. Am. J. Otol. 7: 350–353 (1986).

12 Sadé, J.; Luntz, M.; Wolfson, S.; Berger, G.: The infant's pre-tympanic region of the eustachian tube in health and disease. Int. J. ped. Otorhinolar. 10: 237–243 (1985).

13 Sadé, J.; Wolfson, S.; Luntz, M.; Berger, G.: The anatomical regions of the eustachian tube; in Sadé, The eustachian tube, pp. 31–40 (Kugler, Amsterdam 1987).

14 Berger, G.; Sadé, J.; Sachs, Z.; Luntz, M.: The involvement of the eustachian tube mucosal lining in acute and secretory otitis media; in Sadé, The eustachian tube, pp. 55–61 (Kugler, Amsterdam 1986).

15 Zöllner, F.: Anatomie, Physiologie and Klinik der Ohrtrompete (Springer, Berlin 1942).
16 Sadé, J.: Pathology and pathogenesis of serous otitis media. Archs Otolar. *84:* 297–305 (1966).
17 Sadé, J.; Halevy, A.; Hadas, E.: Clearance of middle ear effusions and middle ear pressures. Ann. Otol. Rhinol. Lar. *85:* suppl. 25, pp. 58–62 (1976).
18 Kitajiri, N.; Hashida, Y.; Sando, I.; Doyle, W.J.: Histopathology of otitis media in infants with cleft and high-arched palates. Ann. Otol. Rhinol. Lar. *94:* 44–50 (1985).
19 Zechner, G.: Auditory tube and middle ear mucosa in nonpurulent otitis media. Ann. Otol. Rhinol. Lar. *89:* suppl. 68, pp. 87–90 (1980).

J. Sadé, MD, Department of Otolaryngology, Meir Hospital,
Kfar Saba 44 281 (Israel)

Adv. Oto-Rhino-Laryng., vol. 39, pp. 37–43 (Karger, Basel 1988)

Pathophysiological Aspects of Vestibular Disorders

C.R. Pfaltz

Department of Otorhinolaryngology, University of Basel, Switzerland

Man has the capability of controling posture and motion in relation to his surroundings. This is achieved by reflex and voluntary control systems the responses of which are based on sensory information received from: (1) the vestibular end organs; (2) visual afferents, and (3) somatosensory perception. These three sensory systems are the basis of the *balance system*.

In the following I should like to discuss two typical disorders of the balance system which are caused by a deficient coordination of visual, somatosensory and vestibular sensory input: motion sickness and vestibular compensation following unilateral lesions.

Motion Sickness

Kinetosis or motion sickness refers to the syndrome of dizziness, perspiration, nausea, vomiting, increased salivation, yawning and generalized malaise caused by excessive stimulation of the vestibular system. The primary cause of motion sickness is motion, although many stimuli (visceral, psychic, visual) may contribute to its incidence [7]. The aetiology of motion sickness is still discussed. The hypothesis of *vestibular overstimulation* is no longer valid and the alternative, more acceptable explanation of the essential cause of this disorder rests on behaviourable evidence which suggests that the condition must be viewed, not as an isolated vestibular phenomenon, but as the response of the organism to discordant motion cues [3]. The importance of conflicting sensory cues (sensory conflict theory) as the principal aetiological factor is now widely accepted and known as *the neural mismatch or sensory rearrangement theory* [17]. However, it has to be emphasized that the conflict is not just between signals from the vestibular apparatus, the eyes, and other receptors stimulated by forces acting on the body, but that these signals are also at variance with those which the central nervous system *expects* to receive [3]. In normal locomotor activity disturbances of body movement, such as when one is pushed or unexpectedly trips, are typically brief and the *mismatch* between the *actual* and the *expected* sensory input from the body's motion detectors is employed to initiate corrective motor responses. However, if there is a sustained change in the sensory input due, for example, to environmental factors or disease, then the continued presence of a high level of neural mismatch indicates to the central nervous system that the 'internal model' is in error.

Essential to the *sensory conflict* or *neural mismatch theory* of motion sickness is that the presence of a sustained mismatch signal of sufficient intensity has two effects: (1) it produces a modification of the internal model, and (2) it evokes the sequence of neuro-vegetative responses characterizing the motion sickness syndrome [3].

It has been demonstrated that cortical areas, vision and gastrointestinal impulses are not required to produce motion sickness. Recent reports indicate that also the cerebellum and the chemoreceptor trigger zone are no longer considered essential. The *vestibular receptors* and *nuclei*, the reticular system and the vomiting centre in the brain stem appear to be the essential structures in the development of the motion sickness syndrome. The maintenance of balance between the acetylcholine and the norepinephrine activity in the vestibular and the reticular neurons during vestibular stimulation appears to be responsible for the development of motion sickness and the *habituation* to it [18].

Vestibular Compensation

Functional recovery after unilateral vestibular lesions is mostly referred to as *'vestibular compensation'*. The central nervous system (CNS) should execute 2 major tasks: (1) Re-establishment of balance, by reducing or abolishing the static asymmetry in the postural tone of skeletal and eye muscles. Once re-established, head and body tilt as well as ocular nystagmus will be absent. (2) Recalibration of the gain of dynamic vestibular reflexes in order to assure symmetrical compensatory vestibulospinal and vestibulo-ocular reflex (VOR) action during motion of the body and head [15].

Recent animal experiments [5] show that vestibular compensation is a goal-directed process, induced by the system's functional error and directed to its elimination. Initiation, maintenance and formation rate of the neural modifications responsible for vestibular compensation depend on the error signal, i.e. the asymmetrical input signal. The phenomenon of functional restoration appears to be the result of specific control mechanisms that guide adaptive changes, including recovery processes in the adult CNS.

Prognosis of functional restoration, either by recovery or by compensation, depends primarily on the site of the lesion, secondly on its pathogenesis and last but not least on the general functional state of the patient's CNS. Cerebral arteriosclerosis and senile degenerative encephalopathy, involving the brain stem, generally cause a substantial delay of either spontaneous recovery or central compensation of vestibular lesions [11,12].

Motion of the head or motion of the visual surroundings will result in loss of sight of a previously stationary visual target. At the same time it will induce some sort of spatial disorientation, unless compensatory eye movements cancel these unwanted subjective sensations. This is achieved by both optokinetic and VOR mechanisms. The two systems are intimately coupled and the common output of the optokinetic system (OKS) and the vestibular system (VS) subserve the maintenance of equilibrium and maintenance in space. The degree of functional disorders of one or both sensorimotor systems will depend on the site of the lesion and on their structural organization [15].

The close cooperation between the visual and the vestibular systems during eye-head coordinated gaze movements following the movement of objects in space, is of fundamental importance with regard to central compensation of uni- and bilateral vestibular loss of function [14]. For these parts of the optokinetic system and the pursuit system (PS) which are not influenced by the vestibular system, a pathological VOR will sucessfully be compensated by the OKS and the PS as long as the lesion is strictly confined to the peripheral vestibular neuron. If, however, a lesion impairs the pathways commonly used by both the VS and the OKS, i.e. those connecting the vestibular nuclei with the subcortical gaze and oculomotor centres, the coordinated functions of the PS, OKS and the VOR will inevitably break down. Pathological vestibular signals will lead to gaze errors, causing contradictory erroneous information about spatial orientation. This conflicting situation, which is neither suppressed nor eliminated, may thus impede the compensation of the vestibular disorder by the visual system [12].

Vestibular disorders following the removal of an acoustic schwannoma are not only due to the sudden postoperative loss of peripheral vestibular function but sometimes also to the pre-operative compression of the brain stem and/or the cerebellum as well as to an intraoperative damage to these anatomical structures. From a hypothetical point of view the time course and mode of vestibular compensation after acoustic neuroma surgery will therefore be quite different from the one observed after labyrinthectomy or vestibular neurectomy.

In the present study we have made an attempt to investigate the pathophysiological factors influencing the course of central vestibular compensation after acoustic neuroma surgery in a series of 10 patients who have been followed up closely for a period of at least 6 months up to 2 years, before and after removal of a Schwannoma of the vestibular nerve.

Vestibular compensation following the surgical removal of an VIIIth nerve Schwannoma is achieved by means of a multisensory process, requiring 'a fully balanced supravestibular control' [6]. Any defect in sensory input or central nervous structure delays functional restoration when occurring during the early stages of compensation [8].

According to animal experiments [16] functional recovery following unilateral lesions of the vestibular end-organ or peripheral neuron occurs fast, i.e. at about the time when spontaneous nystagmus has disappeared (days 4–5) and is accomplished by day 10 postoperatively. After acoustic neuroma surgery vestibular compensation is achieved on the average after 4 weeks to 2 months, depending less on the age of the patient than on the functional state of his CNS. OKR tests are of prognostic importance because OKN disorders indicate brain stem and/or cerebellar lesions involving the system of eye-head coordination. In acoustic neuroma patients central compensation is delayed considerably, because visual circuits underlying OKR are not able to substitute for the vestibular defects, and because vestibular and visual circuits share common pathways which are not functioning normally.

We have learned from animal experiments [8] that an early critical period exists during which adaptive changes in the vestibular system can be induced by multisensory inputs. During recent years we have made several attempts to study these adaptive changes and their influences on the OKR and the VOR with special reference to mechanisms related to visual-vestibular interaction [13]. We were able to demonstrate a visual-vestibular transfer mechanism which is offering some practical therapeutic consequences with respect to the rehabilitation of unilateral vestibular functional disorders: OK or combined vestibular OK training in cases of unilateral vestibular dysfunction may assist to improve the gain of the OKR and the VOR on the side of the lesion more rapidly than without training, and lead to the gradual elimination of the asymmetric input signal [10]. These findings emphasize the importance of an early multisensory training of the acoustic neuroma patient, starting – if possible – not later than the 5th postoperative day. It should not only consist of active and passive head and body exercises (4 + 9) but also of an OK training in order to improve the gain of the impaired VOR dynamics, i.e. the gain of the vestibular responses corresponding with the side of the lesion [13].

Conclusions

The vestibular, visual and proprioceptive system represent the sensorimotor basis of upright position and gait. Action potentials, elicited by adequate physical stimuli at the level of the mechanoreceptors of the vestibular endorgan, provide the necessary information which is indispensable for a continuous spatial orientation. The convergence of the three sensory systems in the brain stem is not only the basis of physiologic static and locomotion, but also under pathologic conditions contributes to the restoration of upright position and gait by achieving central compensation of peripheral vestibular dysfunction. Compensation is a goal-directed process, induced by the system's functional error and directed to its elimination. The *asymmetrical input* resulting from a peripheral vestibular lesion, can be systematically modified by subsequently exposing the subject to various accelerative and gravitational forces or – using the transfer mechanism of *habituation* – by repeated optokinetic stimulation. Initiation, maintenance and formation rate of the neural modifications responsible for compensation depend on the *error signal,* i.e. the *asymmetrical input signal.* Vestibular compensation and probably also vestibular habituation appear to be the result of specific control mechanisms, guiding adaptive changes. The underlying neurophysiological mechanisms of central vestibular compensation seem to be closely related to those of vestibular habituation. They depend on neural networks, built up by modifiable components and capable of learning. They have to serve multisensory purposes because in the case of vestibular compensation functional integration of multisensory inputs are needed which tonically and dynamically substitute for the missing peripheral vestibular signals. In this multisensory substitution process the remaining intact vestibular endorgan appears particularly involved in creating the dynamic counterpart. The earlier multisensory information is provided the better adapted the recalibration of gain will be and the better the final compensation [16]. Vestibular compensation requires an actively behaving subject. It resembles a sensorimotor learning process implicating the concerted activity of many integrated nervous structures. By means of the convergence of vestibulo-visual information conditioned compensatory oculo- and locomotor responses are developed. They counteract or suppress inadequate or pathologic vestibular responses. Thus, contradictory vestibular, visual and proprioceptive information can be eliminated, which might interfere with spatial orientation and result in the typical symptoms of a disturbed equilibrium.

References

1   Allum, J.H.J.: Organization of stabilizing reflex responses in tibialis anterior muscles following ankle flexion perturbations of standing man. Brain Res. *264:* 297–301 (1983).
2   Allum, J.H.J.; Pfaltz, C.R.: Postural control in man following acute unilateral peripheral vestibular deficit. Proc. Symp. on Vestibular and Visual Control of Posture and Locomotor Equilibrium, Houston 1983.
3   Benson, A.J.: Motion sickness; in Dix, Hood, Vertigo, pp. 391–426 (Wiley, Chichester 1984).
4   Dix, M.R.: The rationale and technique of head exercises in the treatment of vertigo. Acta oto-rhino-lar. belg. *33:* 370–384 (1979).
5   Flohr, H.; Lacour, M.; Kaga, K.; Precht, W.; Pfaltz, C.R.: Panel discussion synthesis: neurophysiological and diagnostic aspects of vestibular compensation. Adv. Oto-Rhino-Laryng., vol. 30, pp. 319–329 (Karger, Basel 1983).
6   Jeannerod, M.; Courgon, J.H.; Flaudrin, J.M.; Schmid, R.: Supravestibular control of vestibular compensation after hemilabyrinthectomy in the cat; in Lesion-induced neuronal plasticity in sensori motor systems, pp. 208–220 (Springer, Berlin 1981).
7   Johnson, W.H.; Jongkees, L.B.W.: Motion sickness; in Kornhuber, Handbook of sensory physiology, pp. 389–404 (Springer, Berlin 1974).
8   Lacour, M.: Neurophysiological and diagnostic aspects of vestibular compensation. Neurophysiological and clinical aspects of vestibular compensation. Adv. Oto-Rhino-Laryng., vol. 30, pp. 319–329 (Karger, Basel 1983).
9   Norre, M.E.; Weerdt, W. de: Principe et élaboration d'une technique de rééducation vestibulaire, le 'vestibular training'. Annls. Oto-lar. *96:* 217–227 (1969).
10 Pfaltz, C.R.: Vestibular habituation and central compensation. Adv. Oto-Rhino-Laryng., vol. 22, p. 136 (Karger, Basel 1977).

11 Pfaltz, C.R.; Meran, A.: Sudden unilateral loss of vestibular function. Adv. Oto-Rhino-Laryng., vol. 27, p. 159 (Karger, Basel 1981).

12 Pfaltz, C.R.; Boehmer, A.: The influence of the pursuit and optokinetic system upon vestibular responses in man. Acta oto-lar. 91: 515–520 (1981).

13 Pfaltz, C.R.: Vestibular compensation. Physiological and clinical aspects. Acta oto-lar. 95: 402–406 (1983).

14 Pfaltz, C.R.; Allum, J.H.J.: Vestibular compensation after acoustic neuroma surgery. Adv. Oto-Rhino-Laryng., vol. 34, pp. 164–175 (Karger, Basel 1984).

15 Pfaltz, C.R.: Interaction of the vestibulo-ocular and the optokinetic reflex. Recent development in ORL, pp. 110–113 (Budapest 1984).

16 Precht, W.: Neurophysiological and diagnostic aspects of vestibular compensation. Adv. Oto-Rhino-Laryng., vol. 30, pp. 319–329 (Karger, Basel 1983).

17 Reason, J.T.: Motion sickness adaptation. A neural mismatch model. J. R. Soc. Med. 71: 819–829 (1978).

18 Wood, C.D.; Manno, J.E.; Wood, M.J.; Manno, B.R.; Redetzki, H.M.; Mims, M.E.: Mechanisms of medications and motion sickness. Proc. 7th Int. Man in Space Symp., Houston 1986.

Prof. Dr. C.R. Pfaltz, Department of Otorhinolaryngology,
University of Basel, CH–4031 Basel (Switzerland)

Adv. Oto-Rhino-Laryng., vol. 39, pp. 44–51 (Karger, Basel 1988)

Vertigo Caused by Disorders of the Cervical Vertebral Column

Diagnosis and Treatment

E. Biesinger

Department of Otorhinolaryngology, University of Tübingen, Tübingen, FRG

Introduction

Physicians practicing chiropractics are well acquainted with the correlation between cervical spine pathology and neuro-otological symptoms such as tinnitus, vertigo, neuralgia and sudden hearing loss. The treatment of cervical spinal disease therefore plays an important role in modern neuro-otological practice.

Due to the detailed research of De Kleijn and Nienwentruyse [3], De Jong [2], Decher [1], Jongkees [7], Hülse [6], Reker [13], Ryan and Cope [14] and others, much more is now known about the connection between the vestibular system and the muscular receptors (proprioreceptors) of the cervical vertebral column.

Pathogenesis

On reviewing the literature one can find three main possible origins of the cervical vertigo: (1) a participation of the sympathetic nerve system; (2) a vascular origin, caused by disorders of the vertebral artery, and (3) a participation of the proprioreceptors of the upper cervical spine, caused by pure functional disorders in the segments C0–C2.

Generally, the symptom vertigo alone does not allow an instant assumption of one of these pathological occurrences.

What are the clinical findings indicating that vertigo is caused by disorders of the cervical vertebral column?

History

The following symptoms described by patients lead to the diagnosis of 'cervical vertigo': (1) when patients have complaints in the cervical region, especially following trauma; (2) when the vertigo can be provoked by certain positionings or movements of the head; (3) when the duration of vertigo is short (seconds) and the intensity of vertigo decreases: this vertigo of short duration is provoked by certain positionings of the head, the other vertigo type, of a longer duration, indicates stenosis of the vertebral artery [6].

Clinical Examination of the Cervical Vertebral Column

Clinical examination of the cervical vertebral column includes the clinical inspection of posture, the palpation of muscles and ligaments and the examination of the range of movement.

Inspection of Posture

According to Kapandji [8], the head is correctly balanced on the cervical vertebral column when the cervical lordosis has its vertex in the projection of C4 (fig. 1). Deviations in this ideal posture lead to a functional imbalance of the head and cervical spine, creating uneven compression on the articulation surfaces of the first three vertebrae and unequal tension on bones, ligaments and muscles. This disturbance of the joint function diminishes the range of motion.

Thus, the clinical finding is a lack of mobility in the first three vertebral segments. An excessive cervical lordosis is a typical finding in all patients with cervical vertigo. Figure 2 shows that every variation from the normal posture will disturb the balance in the lever system of the head and neck.

Palpation

Pain in the suboccipital region is a reaction of the muscular system, caused by straining of the vertebral joints. Therefore, a thorough examination should be done on the basis of specific muscle tests to determine the extent of weakness or shortening of the muscles [10].

Testing the Mobility of the Cervical Vertebral Column

A vertebral dysfunction can only be diagnosed by palpation between the individual vertebrae during cervical movement [12]. Testing the range of motion of the cervical vertebral column as a whole is not sufficient, as

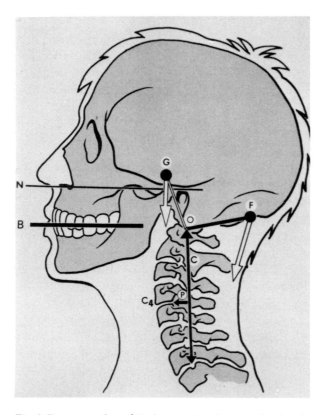

Fig. 1. Demonstration of the lever system between head and cervical vertebral column [8]: the fulcrum O lies at the level of the occipital condyles; the force G is produced by the weight of the head applied through its centre of gravity lying near the sella turcica; the force F is produced by the posterior neck muscles which constantly counter balance the weight of the head.

the proprioreceptors of the first three segments are combined with the vestibular system. While palpation of the segments during mobility is not easy to learn, special courses are offered by various chiropractic schools.

X-Ray Examination
According to Wackenheim [15] and Gutmann [5], X-rays of the cervical vertebral column not only show the morphological findings but also aspects which give more information about its function and posture. Therefore, as shown in figures 3–8, the description of X-ray contents

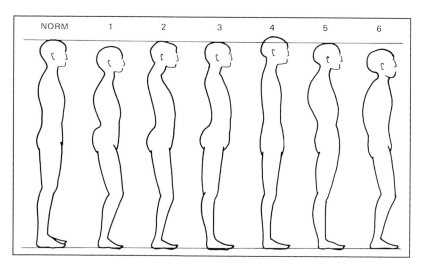

Fig. 2. Any faulty posture creates a dysbalance of the lever system between the head and the cervical vertebral column [11].

should depict congenital disorders or degenerative changes as well as the posture and position of the vertebrae. Thus, both the X-ray and clinical findings together are the elements of diagnosis and therapy.

The basic X-ray examinations are of antero-posterior and lateral projections. In some cases X-rays taken obliquely (of possible intervertebral foramina stenosis), X-rays taken in maximal flection and deflection of the head (of possible instability of the vertebrae), and tomography and computerized tomography are required.

Considering the clinical and functional findings, X-ray examinations may show three typical situations in patients with cervical vertigo:

(1) Clinical examinations showing functional disorders in the segments C0/C1. The X-ray (fig. 3) confirming this finding by showing rotation between the atlas and the axis or (fig. 4) excessive lordosis of the cervical spine.

(2) Clinical examinations showing functional disorders of cervical vertebral joints. The X-ray demonstrating changes resulting from a trauma like incomplete growth of two vertebrae (fig. 5) or degenerative changes with arthrosis of the uncovertebral joints (fig. 6).

(3) Clinical examinations showing functional disorders and the X-ray showing rare congenital disorders like a basilar invagination (fig. 7) which

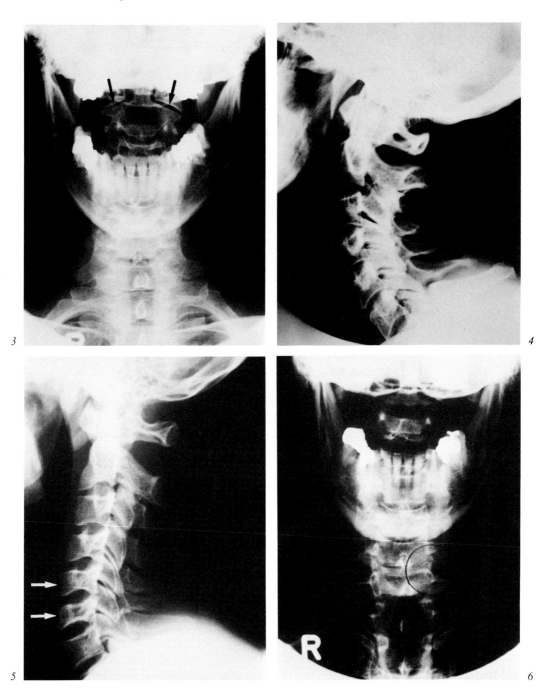

3

4

5

6

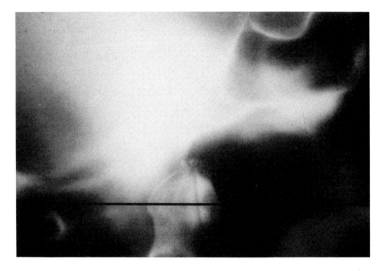

7

Fig. 3. Asymmetry of the at-
lantoaxial interspaces indicates a
rotated position of the atlas.

Fig. 4. Excessive lordosis of
the cervical vertebral column.

Fig. 5. Compression of vertebrae C5 and C6 due to trauma in
childhood.

Fig. 6. Arthrosis of the uncovertebral joint C6/C7.

Fig. 7. Basilar invagination:
The odontoid tip lies 8 mm above
the palatooccipital line (Chamber-
lain's line).

Fig. 8. Hypoplasia of the
posterior arch of the atlas.

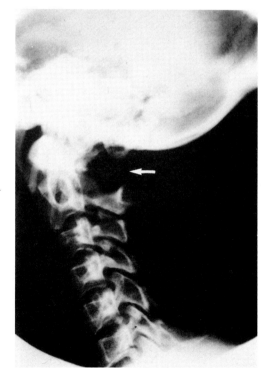

8

can cause vertigo and labyrinthine complaints [4], or a dysplasia of the dorsal arch of atlas (fig. 8).

Finally, after combining clinical examinations and X-ray studies there are two possible diagnoses: (1) vertigo with pure functional disorders of the cervical vertebral column, or (2) vertigo with functional disorders and degenerative findings or congenital disorders of the cervical vertebral column.

Therapy

Adequate physiotherapy is required, including the correction of the functional problems of the entire vertebral column, the stretching of shortened muscles and the strengthening of weak ones in the shoulder and neck region, as well as the mobilization of those joints which show a lack of mobility. It must be emphasized that physiotherapy does not mean massage!

A pure massage removes neither static problems nor dysfunction of the intervertebral joints; on the contrary, the massage leads to an increase of vertigo as the result of mechanical stimulation of the proprioreceptors. The application of ice combined with isometric and isotonic exercises is a very useful method to increase the circulation in the muscles before stretching them. It must also be stressed that the application of ice should never be done alone, but always combined with exercise.

Of course, an experienced physician can treat the patient with chiropractic manipulation of the immobile intervertebral joints. But this manipulation does not treat the cause itself: the faulty alignment of the vertebral column. Therefore, good physiotherapy is better done before manipulation to restore the normal posture. In some cases, careful infiltration with local anaesthetics into the short neck muscles can be effective.

Discussion

Vertigo caused by the cervical vertebral column is mainly due to functional disorders, especially of the first two intervertebral joints. The diagnostic steps and the typical findings are described. The most important findings in nearly all cases is the excessive lordosis of the cervical vertebral column as a result of faulty alignment. Therefore, good physiotherapy should be the first step in treating the patient, combined with chiropractic manipulation or local anaesthesia if necessary. Of special importance is physiotherapy in those cases, where X-ray examinations show degenerative or congenital disorders of the cervical vertebral column.

It is recommendable that otolaryngologists work together with a well-educated physiotherapist. In countries where German is spoken, a good education for physiotherapists should include a further education in manual therapy and functional anatomy according to Klein-Vogelbach [11].

In only a few cases is disturbance of the vertebral artery by skeletal disorders the reason for vertigo. The future will reveal if operating a stenosis of the vertebral artery according to Kehr and Jung [9] will be successful.

References

1 Decher, H.: Die zervikalen Syndrome in der Hals- Nasen- Ohren-Heilkunde (Thieme, Stuttgart 1969).
2 De Yong, J.M.V.B.: Over cervicale Nystagmus en aanverwante verschijnselen; Academic Thesis, Amsterdam (1967).
3 De Kleijn, A.; Nienwentruyse, A.C.: Schwindelanfälle und Nystagmus bei einer bestimmten Stellung des Kopfes. Acta oto-lar. *11:* 55 (1927).
4 Elies, W.; Plester, D.: Basiläre Impression. Eine Differentialdiagnose des Morbus Menière. Archs Otolar. *106:* 232 (1980).
5 Gutmann, G.: Funktionelle Pathologie und Klinik der Wirbelsäule, vol. I/1 (Fischer, Stuttgart 1979).
6 Hülse, M.: Die zervikalen Gleichgewichtsstörungen (Springer, Berlin 1983).
7 Jongkees, L.B.W.: Cervical vertigo. Laryngoscope *79:* 1473 (1969).
8 Kapandji, I.A.: The physiology of the joints, vol. 3 (Churchill Livingstone, Edinburgh 1974).
9 Kehr, P.; Jung, A.: Chirurgie der Arteria vertebralis an den Bewegungssegmenten der Halswirbelsäule; in Gutmann, Funktionelle Pathologie und Klinik der Wirbelsäule, vol. 1, Teil 4 (Fischer, Stuttgart 1985).
10 Kendall, F.P.; Kendall, E.: Muscles, testing and function (Williams & Wilkins, Baltimore 1983).
11 Klein-Vogelbach, S.: Funktionelle Bewegungslehre (Springer, Berlin 1976).
12 Lewitt, K.: Manuelle Medizin (Urban & Schwarzenberg, München 1978).
13 Reker, U.: Leistung der Propriozeptoren der Halswirbelsäule beim zerviko-okulären Reflex. HNO *33:* 424 (1985).
14 Ryan, G.M.S.; Cope, S.: Cervical vertigo. Lancet *ii:* 1355 (1955).
15 Wackenheim, A.: Roentgen diagnosis of the craniovertebral region (Springer, Berlin 1974).

E. Biesinger, Hals-Nasen-Ohrenklinik der Universität Tübingen, Silcherstrasse 5, D–7400 Tübingen (FRG)

Adv. Oto-Rhino-Laryng., vol. 39, pp. 52–64 (Karger, Basel 1988)

The Surgical Concept for Otosclerosis

Ronald E. Gristwood[1]

Royal Adelaide Hospital, Adelaide, Australia

Otosclerosis: A Continuing Enigma

Although deafness from otosclerosis is a common condition affecting about 1% of the adult white population, and the histological features of the bony lesion in the human labyrinthine capsule and stapes footplate have been extensively studied since it was first described by Politzer [1] in 1893, the cause of otosclerosis nevertheless remains obscure and the factors initiating the histological events are unknown. A familial history of hearing loss in close relatives is obtained in about 50% of the cases, and this finding has supported a supposition of autosomal-dominant inheritance.

Prevalence of Otosclerosis

The prevalence of otosclerosis appears to vary enormously in different racial groups and populations. It is generally established that otosclerosis is frequent only among Caucasian populations, uncommon in Mongoloid and extremely rare in Negro populations. In two epidemiological investigations [2, 3] into the prevalence of clinical otosclerosis, the rate for females was shown to increase with age from about 6 per 1,000 in the 40- to 49-year age group, to about 9 or 10 per 1,000 in the 50- to 69-year age group. The rate for males was about half that of females. There is no satisfactory explanation of this apparent sex limitation (fig. 1).

[1] The writer wishes to express his indebtedness to Dr. W.N. Venables of the Department of Statistics, University of Adelaide, for statistical analysis of the data.

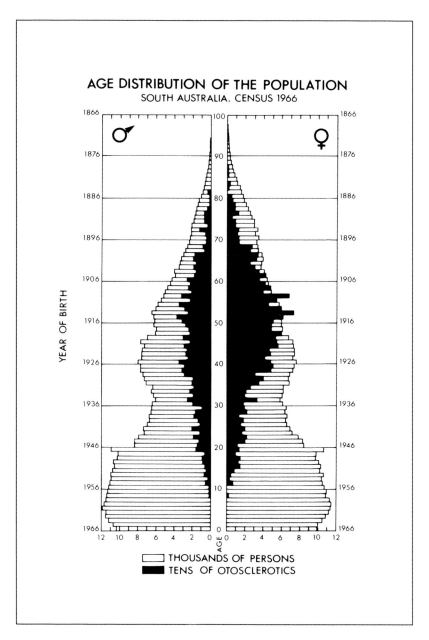

AGE DISTRIBUTION OF THE POPULATION
SOUTH AUSTRALIA, CENSUS 1966

Fig. 1. Surgical cases of otosclerosis in South Australia related to population in 1966 census by age and sex. From Gristwood and Venables [2], courtesy of Editor, *Clinical Otolaryngology.*

Age of Onset of Hearing Loss

The factors determining the age of onset of hearing loss (and stapedial fixation), which varies widely between puberty and 45 years, are unknown. It is, however, fairly clear that an early age of onset (juvenile otosclerosis) greatly increases the chances of contracting a fulminating lesion with severe and diffuse involvement of the stapes footplate and obliteration of the oval window niche [4]. Unilaterality and minor forms of footplate pathology are associated with a later age of onset.

Classification of the Footplate Lesion

The macroscopic appearance of the otosclerotic focus around the oval window niche and in the stapes footplate can be grouped into several categories of generally increasing severity and surgical difficulty [4]. There seems to be wide variation in the pattern of stapedial footplate pathology between continents and between different regions of the same continent.

An analysis of the footplate findings in 1,013 consecutive surgical cases of stapedial otosclerosis in South Australia is given below.

		Cases	Percent
1	Ligamentous fixation	40	3.9
2	Anterior pole focus (small)	504	49.8
3	Anterior pole focus (large)	37	3.7
4	Posterior pole focus	13	1.3
5	Bipolar foci	52	5.1
6	Marginal obliteration: annular focus	46	4.5
7	Thin biscuit footplate: diffusely opaque	83	8.2
8	Solid, delineated thick biscuit or rice-grain footplate	125	12.3
9	Obliterated footplate and niche	113	11.1

An oval window niche narrowed to less than 0.8 mm due to exostosis of promontory or facial canal or both occurred in 4.1% of the cases. About 25–30% of otosclerotic patients who undergo stapes surgery in Australia have footplates that are grossly and diffusely invaded by otosclerotic bone to become white and thickened. By contrast, the incidence of severe footplate pathology from otosclerosis in Europe and in some parts of the USA is much less.

Author	Country	n	Obliterated %	Solid biscuit, %
Plester*	Germany	1,000	2.3	11.5
Palva*	Finland	250	1.6	5.6
Tos and Barfoed [5]	Denmark	200	1.0	7.5
House*	USA	800	1.2	10.3
Sooy*	USA	5,000	2.0	7.0

* Personal communications 1965–1984.

Sensorineural Loss in Otosclerosis

In many cases of stapedial otosclerosis there is a co-existing sensorineural hearing loss which antedates, develops coincidentally with, or ensues after the conductive hearing impairment. The degree of sensorineural deterioration in otosclerosis may vary in different population groups (and geographical localities). Our experience in South Australia is that the sensorineural deterioration is markedly age-dependent, but much greater than what would be expected from aging processes alone [6] (fig. 2).

Measurements of BC thresholds in otosclerosis are important to estimate the patient's level of sensorineural reserve, and to predict the postoperative hearing level that a patient can expect after surgical correction of a lesion in the transmission system of the middle ear.

The Surgical Concept in Otosclerosis

The treatment of otosclerosis has fascinated otologists for a century. No medical treatment has been proven to be successful. Rehabilitation by means of hearing aids has been paralleled by a variety of surgical procedures devised to by-pass the otosclerotic focus or to replace the fixed ossicle by a mobile one.

The early efforts to improve hearing by stapes mobilization in the latter part of the 19th century were mainly unsuccessful because of limited access through an incision in the tympanic membrane and inadequate instrumentation, illumination and magnification.

Fenestration of the lateral semicircular canal was developed in multiple stages by Sourdille [7] of France, and in one stage by Lempert [8] of the

magnitude of surgical trauma, from whatever cause, is directly related to the incidence of irreversible damage to the membraneous labyrinth and its contents. Small openings in the stapes footplate have less chance of causing labyrinthine injury than operations of total footplate removal. In recent years, techniques that create small footplate fenestras have found increasing favour.

Stapedotomy techniques, which create a small calibrated opening in the post-central area of the footplate, using needles, microhooks, microburrs or lasers, of necessity require some type of solid piston prosthesis to establish the sound-conductive mechanism. These piston prostheses are made of Teflon, stainless steel, Teflon steel or Teflon platinum and vary in diameter from 0.3, 0.4, 0.5, 0.6 and 0.8 mm.

Pistons can be used with or without an intervening tissue graft. The author's preference is to seal the oval window niche with a connective tissue graft placed as a collar surrounding the piston.

Post-Operative Outcome of Stapedectomy

I should like to present the long-term results of stapedectomy using piston techniques. The cases reported are consecutive and therefore unselected, and have been grouped according to: (a) footplate pathology, and (b) age at operation (50 years and under, and those over 50 years). The numbers followed up, the means of the AC thresholds, the mean bone-air gaps, together with standard deviations and confidence intervals at various post-operative times over a 10-year period are given for 579 thin footplates fixed by an anterior pole focus of otosclerosis, and for 142 obliterative cases.

Thin Footplates

In the 579 consecutive cases of thin footplates the overall results are much better in the age group 50 years and under in that: (i) the mean AC levels (0.5, 1 and 2 kHz) are stable over 10 years and about 10 dB better than in the over 50s ($p < 10^{-6}$); (ii) the mean bone-air gap (0.5, 1 and 2 kHz) is consistently overclosed in reference to pre-operative BC thresholds ($p < 10^{-3}$); (iii) the standard deviations are smaller at 11–13 dB.

In those over 50 years of age the standard deviations are slightly greater at 14–15 dB, and the bone-air gaps become slightly positive after 5 years, this being almost certainly a presbyacusis effect. Because pre-

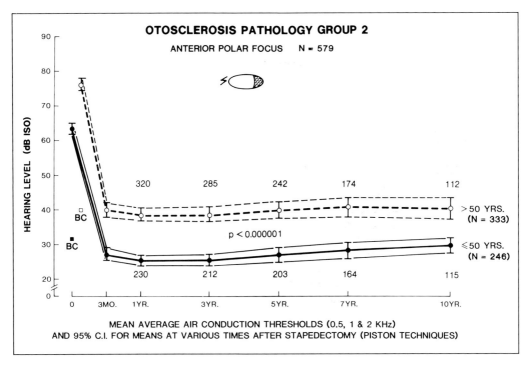

Fig. 3. Mean air conduction responses after stapedectomy for type 2 footplate pathology. Reproduced from Gristwood [6].

operative BC measurements are used as the basis of assessing the bone-air gap it will be appreciated that any apparent increase in the mean bone-air gap post-operatively can be due to either conductive or sensorineural losses or both (fig. 3; table I).

When data are distributed in an approximately Gaussian form, as here, the formula (mean + 1 SD) gives the 84th percentile. In those 50 years and under, 84% attained closure of the bone-air gap to within 8.6 dB at 5 years and to within 10 dB at 10 years. In the over 50s, 84% attained closure to within 16 dB at 5 and 10 years. Thus, while the aggregate results for piston techniques after partial stapedectomy for anterior polar otosclerosis are highly satisfactory in the short and long term, there is a very obvious benefit for the age group 50 years and under whether assessed by mean air conduction thresholds or by mean bone-air gaps.

Table I. Mean bone-air gaps (0.5–2 kHz) after stapedectomy for 579 cases of type 2 foot-plate pathology: reproduced from Gristwood [6]

Pathology group 2: anterior pole focus
Sample size: 579

Age group	Observation time	Number	Mean	SD	95% CI for mean
≤ 50 years	pre-operative BC	246	31.4	11.5	30.0 to 32.9
	pre-operative B/A gap	246	31.9	10.0	30.7 to 33.2
	3-month gap	244	−4.3	10.8	−5.6 to −2.9
	1-year gap	230	−5.3	12.4	−6.9 to −3.7
	3-year gap	212	−5.2	12.3	−6.9 to −3.5
	5-year gap	203	−4.1	12.7	−5.8 to −2.3
	7-year gap	164	−1.7	14.1	−3.9 to 0.5
	10-year gap	115	−1.5	11.4	−3.6 to 0.6
> 50 years	pre-operative BC	333	39.8	13.6	38.4 to 41.3
	pre-operative B/A gap	333	36.3	10.6	35.1 to 37.4
	3-month gap	330	0.1	14.1	−1.5 to 1.6
	1-year gap	320	−1.0	14.5	−2.6 to 0.6
	3-year gap	284	−1.2	14.3	−2.9 to 0.5
	5-year gap	242	0.7	15.0	−1.2 to 2.6
	7-year gap	174	2.9	14.5	0.7 to 5.0
	10-year gap	112	4.1	12.0	1.9 to 6.4

Obliterative Cases

Analysis of 142 consecutive cases of obliterative otosclerosis after obligatory small hole fenestras and piston techniques shows post-operative results that are less impressive than those for thin footplates. Both age groups in the obliterative series have small positive bone-air gaps of about 4–5 dB in the first 5 years after surgery. Differences between age groups are not statistically significant until 10 years after surgery when paradoxically, the older group had an advantage over the younger (p < 10^{-2}). The mean AC threshold levels (0.5, 1 and 2 kHz) are significantly better in the younger age group during the first 3 post-operative years, after which there is no detectable difference between age groups (table II, fig. 4). These findings led us to question whether small hole fenestras are inferior to medium and large hole fenestras as indeed one might suppose on the basis of the difference in outcome in the two categories of footplate pathology.

Table II. Mean bone-air gaps (0.5–2 kHz) after stapedectomy for 142 cases of obliterative oval window otosclerosis: reproduced from Gristwood [6]

Pathology groups 9 and 10: obliterated oval window Sample size: 142					
Age group	Observation time	Number	Mean	SD	95% CI for mean
≤ 50 years	Pre-operative BC	68	34.4	17.1	30.3 to 38.6
	Pre-operative B/A gap	68	38.2	9.9	35.8 to 40.6
	3-month gap	68	4.9	15.8	1.0 to 8.7
	1-year gap	64	5.6	16.8	1.4 to 9.8
	3-year gap	61	4.0	15.2	0.1 to 7.9
	5-year gap	60	4.4	16.6	0.2 to 8.7
	7-year gap	51	8.6	18.1	3.6 to 13.7
	10-year gap	37	9.9	17.2	4.1 to 15.6
> 50 years	pre-operative BC	74	48.0	16.2	44.2 to 51.8
	Pre-operative B/A gap	74	41.2	8.8	39.1 to 43.2
	3-month gap	74	3.8	12.4	0.9 to 6.6
	1-year gap	72	3.5	13.3	0.4 to 6.7
	3-year gap	65	2.0	14.6	−1.7 to 5.6
	5-year gap	61	1.7	12.9	−1.6 to 5.0
	7-year gap	49	4.7	13.9	0.7 to 8.7
	10-year gap	37	2.5	13.4	−1.9 to 7.0

Effect of Hole Size and Piston Diameter

To study this problem further, we analysed the effect of size of fenestra (small, medium and large) and diameter of piston (0.6 and 0.8 mm) on 576 cases of thin stapes footplates fixed by an anterior polar focus of otosclerosis (because numbers were adequate and technical difficulties were rare in that category), all operated on by one and the same surgeon [6].

Footplate fenestra	Piston diameter		
	0.6 mm	0.8 mm	totals
Small	105	26	131
Medium	182	173	355
Large	36	54	90
Totals	323	253	576

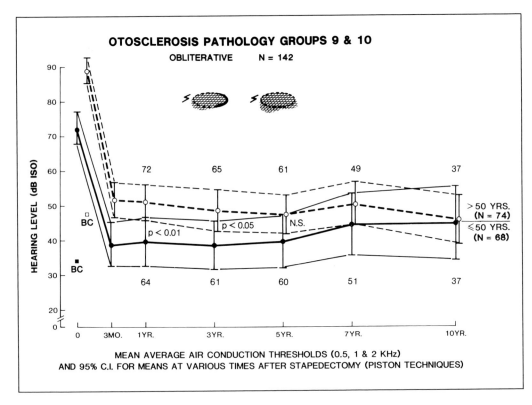

Fig. 4. Mean air conduction responses after stapedectomy for obliterative oval window otosclerosis. Reproduced from Gristwood [6].

There is some evidence that the slimmer the diameter of the piston prosthesis the less efficient it is at closing the bone-air gap for low frequencies. Patients who had a medium hole and a thick piston (0.8 mm) or in any case a piston adapted to the size of the fenestra, tended to have a very slight long-term advantage with a slightly smaller mean bone-air gap (0.5–2 kHz) compared to others. In particular, it was evident that a large size of footplate fenestra should be avoided if at all possible in piston techniques. Hole size and piston diameter and their interactions accounted at most for 5% of the total variation in post-operative outcomes, so prediction is minimal and rigid rules for determining surgical practice cannot be drawn up.

Summary and Conclusions

The aggregate results of the stapedectomy operation for hearing improvement are highly satisfactory in the short and long term when carried out by an experienced and skilled surgeon, using a variety of techniques in carefully selected candidates. An initial bone-air gap of 10 dB or less is achieved in 80–90% of patients. The outcome of stapedectomy is dependent on the patient's level of sensorineural reserve which is age dependent, and on the limitations imposed by stapedial footplate pathology. The advantages of various types of piston prostheses for reconstruction have become increasingly clear. The infrequent complications of immediate and delayed sensorineural losses with impaired speech discrimination are certain to be reduced further in incidence by the increasing adoption of small fenestra techniques with piston prostheses and tissue seals.

There is a definite need for fully informative statistical methods in reporting the results of surgery for hearing improvement if further advances are to be made.

References

1 Politzer, A.: Über primäre Erkrankung der knöchernen Labyrinthkapsel. Z. Ohrenheilk. *25:* 309–327 (1894).
2 Gristwood, R.E.; Venables, W.N.: Otosclerosis in South Australia. Clin. Otolar. *9:* 221–228 (1984).
3 Pearson, R.D.; Kurland, L.T.; Cody, D.T.R.: Incidence of diagnosed clinical otosclerosis. Arch Otolar. *99:* 288–291 (1974).
4 Gristwood, R.E.; Venables, W.N.: A note on progression of the otosclerotic focus. Clin. Otolar. *7:* 257–260 (1982).
5 Tos, M.; Barfoed, C.: Failures and complications in the surgery of otosclerosis. Acta oto-rhino-lar. ital. *2:* 485-493 (1982).
6 Gristwood, R.E.: Deafness from otosclerosis in South Australia; thesis, University of Edinburgh (1981).
7 Sourdille, M.: New technique in surgical treatment of severe and progressive deafness from otosclerosis. Bull. N.Y. Acad. Med. *13:* 673–691 (1937).
8 Lempert, J.: Improvement of hearing in cases of otosclerosis. A new one-stage surgical technic. Archs Otolar. *28:* 42–97 (1938).
9 Shambaugh, G.E., Jr.: Fenestration operation for otosclerosis: experimental investigations and clinical observations in 2,100 operations over a period of 10 years. Acta oto-lary., suppl. 79, pp. 1–101 (1949).
10 Colman, B.H.: Otosclerosis; in Maran, Stell, Clinical otolaryngology, pp. 189–206 (Blackwell, Oxford 1979).

11   Rosen, S.: Mobilization of the stapes to restore hearing in otosclerosis. N. Y. State J. Med. *53:* 2650–2653 (1953).
12   Shea, J.J.: Fenestration of the oval window. Ann. Otol. Rhinol. Lar. *67:* 932–951 (1958).
13   Schuknecht, H.F.: Stapedectomy (Little, Brown, Boston 1971).
14   McGee, T.M.: Techniques and experiences with stapedectomy and metal implant, chap. 39; in Schuknecht, Otosclerosis. Henry Ford Hospital International Symposium, pp. 489–495 (Little, Brown, Boston 1962).

Ronald E. Gristwood, Ch.M., FRCS (Edin.), FRACS, Toynbee House,
12 Walter Street, North Adelaide, South Australia 5006 (Australia)

Adv. Oto-Rhino-Laryng., vol. 39, pp. 65–82 (Karger, Basel 1988)

Advances in Middle Ear Surgery[1]

Klaus Jahnke

Department of Otorhinolaryngology (Head: Prof. Dr. *D. Plester*),
University of Tübingen, FRG

Introduction

In 1970, Plester reported on progress in microsurgery of the ear and
mentioned that otosurgical principles and techniques were undergoing the
most important transformation in their history.

Now, 17 years later, the time has come to see which microsurgical
methods have been *successful,* which have been more or less *abandoned,*
and which have been *recently introduced.* Concepts, techniques, and materials used in reconstructive middle ear surgery are discussed based on our
experience at the Tübingen department; a few unresolved problems are
also mentioned. Often, more than *one* rational operative solution is acceptable. Indications for the individual techniques and materials have been
worked out in long-term studies over the last 15 years.

Myringoplasty is discussed first, followed by ossicular chain reconstruction and treatment of the posterior canal wall in cholesteatoma surgery. In conclusion, a few remarks are made on surgery of otosclerosis and
minor ear malformations.

Myringoplasty

There is not a great deal new to report on myringoplasty. We *underlay*
the perforation with a wet autograft of *temporal fascia* or *tragal perichondrium.* We do not use the overlay technique. Depending on whether an
enaural or retroauricular approach has been selected, small perforations

[1] Supported by the Deutsche Forschungsgemeinschaft, grant Ja/205-8.

can also be closed with *periosteum* from the canal entrance or the mastoid process.

Optimal ingrowth of this abundantly available mesenchymal tissue is encouraged by meticulously *trimming the perforation* and, depending on the size of the defect, *overlapping the transplants* by 2–3 mm. The quilt technique, which Gerlach described in 1972, is well suited for larger perforations in the anterior part of the tympanic membrane. Graft detachment can be avoided by packing the anterior part of the tympanic cavity with antibiotic-soaked *absorbable Gelfoam,* which then drains over the Eustachian tube. Human fibrin adhesive is used for transplant fixation only in exceptional cases, e.g. subtotal defects.

The use of tragal perichondrium with adherent *cartilage* has steadily increased since the mid-1970s. The main indications are atrophic tympanic membrane, absent malleus handle, and Eustachian tube dysfunction. In such cases, the risk of adhesions and retraction pockets is reduced by tragal perichondrium with adherent cartilage. The vibrating capacity of the new drum should be ensured. One advantage which we had observed when using cartilage to prevent the rejection of poorly tolerated porous plastic prostheses was the surprisingly good hearing results achieved with relatively large and cumbersome cartilage grafts.

Temporal fascia or perichondrium should be covered with a *skin flap* from the anterior canal wall in perforations that extend over more than one third of the tympanic membrane diameter, especially perforations located over the Eustachian tube. Such a skin flap should also be used when tympanosclerosis is present, since the frequency of reperforation is higher due to poor local blood supply. The skin of the anterior canal wall is extremely thin and smooth and, therefore, well suited for grafting. We do not advise using retroauricular skin for this indication.

While the indication for application of a *homograft drum* has become stricter, such grafts are, nevertheless, indicated for subtotal defects *with* absent malleus handle. If the stapes footplate is also fixed, a malleovestibulopexy can be performed at a second stage, providing that the middle ear is well ventilated. The formaldehyde-fixed, Cialit-conserved graft should be soaked in water for 24 h before surgery. The new drum is often difficult to distinguish from a normal drum. In a few isolated cases, we still observed rejection reactions several months after surgery. Gluing on the homograft drum with human fibrin adhesive has proved advantageous.

More than 90% of all tympanic membrane perforations can be closed with the techniques mentioned above. Since, with latent dysfunction of tubal ventilation, the risk of retraction pockets and adhesions at the promontory is greater than the risk of reperforation, our patients are asked to perform Valsalva's maneuver as soon after surgery as possible.

In our opinion, there are several disadvantages of the *overlay technique*, i.e. frequent blunting of the anterior tympanomeatal angle and occasional development of an annular cholesteatoma or lateralization of the tympanic membrane. The surgical solution was summarized by Plester and Pusalkar [1981] as follows: With respect to *blunting*, it is important that excessive connective tissue be meticulously trimmed without damaging the epithelium and the lamina propria of the tympanic membrane. The lamina propria of the drum is then completely covered with a free skin flap from the anterior canal wall.

We proceed similarly with *medial auditory canal fibrosis.* This rare disease, the transitional forms of which extend to total atresia of the auditory canal, has only been investigated in the last 15 years. Medial auditory canal fibrosis may be either congenital or the consequence of otitis externa diffusa. Histologic evaluation of excised tissue shows loose fibrous tissue, blood vessels, and small nerves.

The treatment of an *annular cholesteatoma,* a complication of the overlay technique, is relatively simple, providing that the cholesteatoma has not developed too far medially. After meticulous denuding, the matrix attached to the tympanic membrane can be left. A tympanic membrane that has lateralized after the overlay technique is either realigned in the normal position or, if the position is stable, left at the level of the lateral tympanic membrane, and the chain reconstructed with an extra-long columella and an auxiliary ossicle, when necessary.

Ossicular Chain Reconstruction

Opinions on the preferred techniques and materials for reconstruction of the ossicular chain are even more controversial now than in the past. In the early 1970s, most investigators agreed that plastics like polyethylene, because of their relatively high rejection rate, should not be used in surgery of chronic middle ear infections and that only autograft and homograft ossicles or cartilage and, occasionally, steel wire should be used [Plester 1970].

In the mid-1970s, new *porous plastic prostheses* made of polyethylene (Plastipore®) or Teflon partially coated with carbon (Proplast®) were introduced into middle ear surgery. The total ossicular replacement prosthesis (TORPS) and the partial ossicular replacement prosthesis (PORPS) represented a new concept: the ingrowth of connective tissue into the pores was supposed to ensure firm anchorage [Shea et al., 1977]. Clinically, the long-term rejection rate is especially high [Frootko, 1984]: a characteristic crust forms on the prosthesis and eventually grows through the tympanic membrane. Histologically, even in an otherwise infection-free middle ear, the pores of the prosthesis were filled with multinucleated foreign body giant cells, epitheloid cells, and macrophages in various stages of development; blood capillaries were occasionally seen (fig. 1). In 1981, Kerr reported that this material could be phagocytized by macrophages. It, therefore, is not surprising that pronounced foreign body reactions are demonstrable many years later and that the prostheses are eventually rejected. The same holds true for Proplast prostheses. Recently, some ear surgeons have used and recommended new implants made of porous polyethylene (Polycel®). The histocompatibility of these implants, which are produced in a thermal fusion process, is reputed to be better. Since this material was not tested in animals, we implanted it in the bulla tympanica of 8 gerbils. The results were essentially the same (fig. 2) as those obtained with Plastipore prostheses removed from the human middle ear [Cousins and Jahnke, 1987].

The steel wire-reinforced Polycel prostheses, which can be bent to the desired shape during surgery, are reminiscent of a similar technique for cartilage stabilization introduced by Smyth and Kerr in 1967. We suspect that the fate of Polycel implants will be the same as that of other porous plastic implants.

In 1978, the Mainz ENT hospital began using implants of *bioreactive glass ceramic* for reconstruction of the ossicular chain [Reck, 1985] and the Tübingen otorhinolaryngology department, implants of *bioinert aluminum oxide ceramic* [Jahnke and Plester, 1980a, b]. Experimental studies with animals confirmed the excellent biocompatibility of these materials in the middle ear. Bioreactive ceramics are characterized by new bone formation in neighboring tissue due to the escape of ions from the surface of the ceramic material. The term 'bioinert' refers to materials that release no substances into the environment detectable with conventional analytical methods. This definition does not apply to plastics. In addition to aluminum oxide ceramic, the vitreous carbons are also bioinert materials. We also evaluated the suitability of these bioinert materials for middle ear surgery [Jahnke and Schrader, 1984]. *Vitreous carbon* was incorporated in the middle ear of all gerbils without significant signs of irritation (fig. 3). In

Plate I

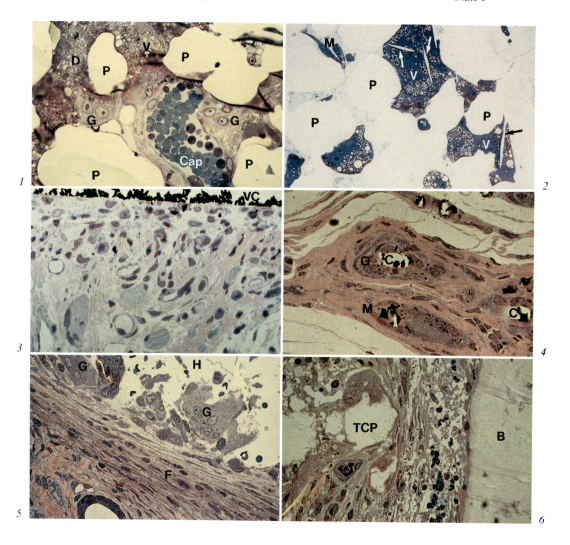

Jahnke

S. Karger, Basel

Fig. 1. Histologic picture of Plastipore prosthesis (P) 4.5 years after implantation; pores filled with foreign body giant cells (G), vacuolated cells (V), debris (D), blood capillary (Cap) as an exceptional finding.

Fig. 2. Light microscopic view of a Polycel footplate prosthesis, 1 month after implantation into the gerbil middle ear. Plastic (P), vacuolated cell (V), macrophage (M), crystalline inclusion (arrow). The pores are rather small.

Fig. 3. Vitreous carbon, 2 months after implantation into the gerbil middle ear. At the implant interface (VC) a loose connective tissue growth with capillary vascularization developed. Cells bordering on the carbon implant do not exhibit degenerative changes or significant stimulation.

Fig. 4. Porous carbon reinforced with carbon fibres 5 months after implantation into the gerbil middle ear. Particles (C) are detached and encapsulated by foreign body giant cells (G) and macrophages (M).

Fig. 5. Histoacryl (H) 12 years after application in the middle ear; note adjacent foreign body giant cells (G) and fibrous capsule (F).

Fig. 6. Porous tricalcium phosphate ceramic (TCP) 5 months after implantation in middle ear of guinea pig; partial replacement by new bone growth (B); no foreign body reaction.

Table I. Ossicular chain reconstruction

---

1   Ossicles (autograft, allograft)
       Malleus head
       Incus
       Stapes (rare, stapes superstructure replacement)
2   Cartilage with perichondrium (autograft)
       Only flat for reinforcement of stapes with classic type III
3   Aluminum oxide ceramic (15–20%)
       One-third hollow shaft implant
       Two-thirds columella
4   Steel wire or plastic band Teflon prosthesis only for malleovestibulopexy or
    stapedectomy

---

contrast to aluminum oxide ceramic, the implant, due to its low wettability, was not covered by mucosa; this material, therefore, is better suited for ventilation tubes or sheeting in adhesion prophylaxis and less suited for ossicular chain reconstruction. Since the foreign body reaction to *porous carbons,* like graphite, pyrolyte carbons, and carbon fiber-reinforced carbons is relatively pronounced (fig. 4), their use in middle ear surgery is not advantageous.

The foreign body reaction can be at least partially explained by the release of carbon particles from the implant surface.

Which materials are best suited for ossicular chain reconstruction? While ceramics should not replace the ossicle bank, these implants do represent an important supplement. Each material has its own indications. Those materials used in Tübingen are listed in table I. In the majority of cases, we transplant *autograft and homograft ossicles,* using the techniques compiled by Plester in 1970. The autograft malleus head is interposed when the location of malleus handle is not too far anterior in relation to the stapes head. Frequently, an incudal body with preserved short crus is used. We consider a homograft stapes indicated in those rare cases with absent stapes superstructure, mobile stapes footplate, and intact incus. The homograft stapes is then transposed with the concave crural side directed toward the promontory and fixed with human fibrin tissue glue. Another indication is a columella with flat tympanic cavity. We seldom use *human fibrin adhesive* for stabilization of the reconstructed chain. The position of the chain should be secured so that adhesive is unnecessary. *Histoacryl,* which was also used in the 1970s as adhesive in the middle ear, has not proved successful, and we do not use it. Minute amounts trigger a foreign body reaction as long as 12 years after implantation (fig. 5).

In summary, the ossicles are well tolerated and have a wide range of applicability. They are particularly cost efficient in Europe because residents are required to remove them as part of their specialist training. Shaping is limited, since the risk of resorption and atrophy is too high. This applies even more to machine-tooled ossicles.

The surface of the ossicles should be drilled as little as possible. Their fit is frequently unstable, and with absent incus and stapes superstructure (i.e. columella must be fashioned), the functional results are often unsatisfactory due to lateralization or fixation at the promontory, Fallopian canal, or lateral attic wall. Obviously, autograft ossicles with adherent cholesteatoma matrix should not be used. The risk of viral infection remains, and transplantation laws in many countries make the use of homograft materials highly problematic.

Utech [1960] was the first to report on the use of cartilage in tympanoplasty. Reconstruction of the sound conduction chain with autograft or homograft *cartilage* columella was repeatedly attempted 15 years ago. The advantages appeared to be easy shaping and low risk of adhesions. Histologic investigations by Steinbach and Pusalkar [1981] and clinical experience, however, clearly showed that, in time, almost all these cartilage grafts failed due to poor blood supply. Hearing impairments usually developed within 3–7 years after surgery. In some cases, the L-shaped cartilage chips fracture. In principle, only cartilage with adherent perichondrium should be used. In our opinion, the only indication in the chain region is the bridging of minute chain defects, e.g. interposition on the stapes head in type III.

We use *bioinert ceramic* in 15–20% of our tympanoplasties and as columella in approximately two-thirds of the cases with absent stapes superstructure, i.e. in those cases with generally unfavorable middle ear pathology. The main indications are as follows: (1) narrow, oval window niche; (2) stapes head close to Fallopian canal; (3) malleus handle far anterior, in relation to stapes, or absent; (4) failure of other materials.

Like bone, ceramic implants must be drilled to the desired shape during surgery with a water-cooled diamond burr. Any sharp edges are smoothed at this time. Before insertion of a columella, the footplate should be covered with a small flap of connective tissue or perichondrium so that the inner ear is protected and, at the same time, a joint-like connection is achieved. Fixation to the Fallopian canal or promontory does not usually occur with this ceramic.

Seating of the hollow shaft prosthesis on the stapes head can be improved by drilling perforations in the distal end and filling them with small connective tissue flaps. Recently, we designed new 'macroporous' implants made of aluminum oxide ceramic which are also available in different lengths (fig. 7). In the hand of an experienced surgeon, these implants are easily drilled in 1–5 min. We recommend estimating the proper length with a 3-mm hook or similar instrument. Another trick is to create a keyhole-shaped notch so that the implant can be securely fitted over the tendon of the stapedius muscle (fig. 8), without risk of fixation to the Fallopian canal like what occurs with ossicles or bioreactive ceramics (fig. 6).

As already mentioned, we frequently use a piece of tragal cartilage with adherent perichondrium to stabilize atrophic tympanic membranes with minimal elasticity. The experience with the palisade technique reported by Heermann and Heermann [1964] also substantiates the suitability of the cartilage graft in this context. Cartilage additionally stabilizes the position of the implant, which, in turn, ensures the width of the tympanic cavity. At present, we use cartilage with most of our ceramic implants, particularly as abutment with absent malleus handle and with unfavorable middle ear ventilation. We sometimes punch a hole in the small cartilage plate to seat the ceramic, which is then encircled by a stable ring of cartilage. Depending on the pathologic conditions in the middle ear, the overall results with ceramic implants are still satisfactory 9 years after surgery. Contraindications are severe inflammation of the middle ear mucosa and obviously poor ventilation of the middle ear. Glass ceramic implants apparently behave similarly. In Mainz, bone pate is used to improve the integration of Ceravital implants at the tympanic membrane. Fixation of the Ceravital implants to the Fallopian canal or the promontory in cases with narrow niches or dislocations can be prevented by coating the Ceravital shaft with bioinert material. Partial disintegration of the material due to repeated infection of the middle ear such as also occurs with ossicles can be prevented by combining Ceravital with a titanium framework [Reck, personal commun.].

With respect to the reconstruction of the ossicular chain with other bioreactive ceramics, the characteristics of hydroxylapatite ceramic implants [Grote, 1984] appear to correspond in many ways to those of Ceravital. Problems arise with regard to bony fixation and partial disintegration in the presence of unfavorable middle ear pathology. The same appar-

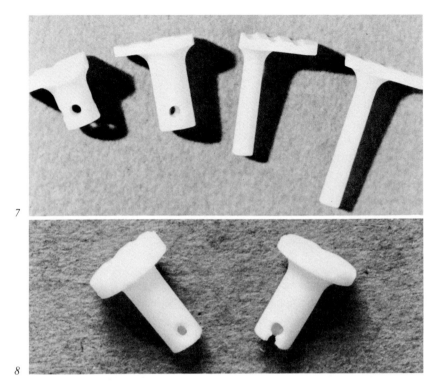

7

8

Fig. 7. Aluminum oxide ceramic implants (Frialit®), L-shaped, for ossicular chain reconstruction, different lengths. The 3- and 5-mm-long hollow-shaft implants with perforations ('macropores') for better anchorage on stapes head; distal end of shaft can also be filled with small pieces of connective tissue.

Fig. 8. 5-mm hollow shaft implants of aluminum oxide ceramic (Frialit®). Left: Implant with intraoperatively drilled perforation; right: implant with keyhole-shaped notch so that it can be securely fitted over tendon of stapedius muscle. Endplates of both implants invested with grooves for insertion of malleus handle.

ently also applies to the bioglass implants which have recently become available on the US market [Merwin, 1986]. These transparent bioglass implants can be shaped with a diamond burr. Direct contact between porous tricalcium phosphate ceramic and bony tissue is necessary before the ceramic can be resorbed and replaced by endogenous bone. This prerequisite is rarely fulfilled in chain reconstruction. Porous tricalcium phosphate ceramic, because of the risk of bony fixation, is also not suited for ossicular chain reconstruction.

We only use steel or platinum *wire,* when necessary, together with a Teflon strut, for malleovestibulopexy or stapedectomy. In addition to minor ear malformations, tympanosclerosis with fixed footplate is another important indication. In such cases, hearing is improved in the second stage since (1) a closed, sterile middle ear, and (2) a stable drum level with guaranteed normal tubal ventilation are necessary. Even though stapedectomy is seldom used for tympanosclerotically fixed footplates, hearing improvement, however, is excellent after this intervention. We prefer cautious preparation of the stapes footplate according to Zöllner [1963]. The choice of operative technique should take the status of the other ear into consideration.

Recently, we saw the following patient who had been treated elsewhere:

A young man with bilateral cholesteatoma had been treated by the creation of a mastoid cavity and then suspension of a steel wire-Teflon prosthesis in the vestibule. A retraction pocket eventually developed which filled with debris and forced the prosthesis deep into the vestibule. The patient became deaf in this ear. A more appropriate approach in this case would have been the creation of a type IV or, if the footplate is fixed, the fitting of a hearing aid.

In the 1980s, the main problem of chain reconstruction is most certainly the fashioning of a columella with absent incus and stapes superstructure. Helms [1983] reported that a sound conduction component of less than 20 dB is achieved in only 30–40% of the cases. These poor results are due to the unfavorable middle ear pathology, which has already destroyed the stapes superstructure, and to the difficulties encountered in stable long-term fixation of the distal end of the transplant or implant to the footplate without injury to the inner ear. The case described above illustrates that the most reliable connection to the vestibule, i.e. a prosthesis suspended by *malleovestibulopexy,* is seldom a viable alternative for surgery of chronic middle ear inflammations. When it is performed, it must be done as a two-stage procedure. Shea and Moretz [1985] introduced a procedure in which, in a second stage, a minute hole is drilled in the footplate to ensure stable anchorage of the pointed distal end of a Plastipore prosthesis. Extravasation of perilymph causes the end of the prosthesis to swell, which, in turn, results in a good connection with the footplate. In our opinion, this solution is also questionable with chronic middle ear inflammations. Our attempts at improving the connection to the footplate include the above-mentioned interposition of mesenchymal tissue. Occasionally, we position a small piece of cartilage with overlapping perichondrium and central bore hole on the footplate. The prosthesis is seated in this hole. Using a similar method, Schobel [personal commun.] implanted a small piece of porous plastic. Recently, the above-mentioned porous plastic prostheses, which have a wire running through the center, have been used. Dislocation of the prosthesis is prevented by a short piece of wire inserted in either a cartilage plate on the footplate or a piece of plastic.

Our experience indicates that the relative vibrations with functioning chain almost never allow the development of a bony connection between ossicle, e.g. incus-columella, and footplate. The contact between a bioreactive ceramic columella and the footplate probably represents a similar situation. We hope to improve the connection between bioinert ceramic columella and footplate by creating macropores on the shaft to encourage the ingrowth of connective tissue.

Another solution to this problem may be two-stage reconstruction of the stapes superstructure. If relative vibrations are absent, a stable bony connection could be achieved by attaching a short homograft ossicle (e.g. stapes with reduced footplate) or an implant of bioreactive ceramic that, however, may not extent to the drum level. Chain reconstruction should then be continued in a second stage. At present, we are testing this procedure in animals. In essence, the aim of middle ear surgery is to give the patient an infection-free ear *with* good hearing in one intervention, when possible.

Cholesteatoma Surgery

In no other area of our specialty are opinions as controversial as in cholesteatoma surgery. The main problem is the treatment of the posterior canal wall. Ten years ago, most ear surgeons preferred the posterior tympanotomy with preservation of the posterior canal wall. Between 1971 and 1972, intact canal wall procedures were used in more than 78% of all first interventions for cholesteatomas in our department. This figure also includes atticotomies with reconstruction of the lateral attic wall. By the end of the 1970s, as Plester reported in 1979 at a congress in Berlin, mastoid cavity construction was being done in almost half of the cases. Today, it is done in more than half of the cases, because long-term studies indicated that, sooner or later, the cholesteatoma recurs in many of those cases with preserved posterior canal wall. These recurrent cholesteatomas are sometimes diagnosed relatively late. Several long-term statistics cited in the literature show a 5-year recurrence rate of 25%. Short-term statistics or data reported in literature that does not cite duration of follow-up and number of reoperations (e.g. control operations) is not relevant for cholesteatomas. Our statistics showed satisfactory short-term results (1-year recurrence rate of less than 4%); the long-term results, however, are far from satisfactory (25% recurrence rate after 10–12 years) [Jahnke et al., 1985]. The decision for an open or a closed technique is based on the individual patient. The important factors to be taken into consideration are as follows: (1) pneumatization of mastoid; (2) extension of cholesteatomas (seldom discernible through antrotomy bore hole); (3) adequate tubal function; (4) age and personality of patient.

The decision can also be influenced during surgery by the probability with which the cholesteatoma matrix can be excised in toto.

The *anteroposterior approach* is indicated in cases with good pneumatization and adequate eustachian tube ventilation; preoperative and intraoperative evaluation of tubal function, however, is often unreliable. Construction of a mastoid cavity is indicated for recurrent cholesteatomas only when recurrence is due to tubal dysfunction. The situation is different when recurrence is attributable to unsatisfactory closure of a defect in the lateral wall of the antrum. Cavity reconstruction is not necessary for well-defined residual cholesteatomas found at reoperation, regardless of whether the intervention is a control operation (i.e. a 'second look') or an operation to improve function. With the rare primary cholesteatomas, the posterior canal wall should, as a rule, be preserved. Informed written consent for reoperation 1 or 2 years after primary surgery should always be obtained from those patients for whom the anteroposterior approach is to be used. Due to the high long-term recurrence rate in patients under the age of 20, reoperation should be the rule rather than the exception in this age group. In our opinion, this also applies for temporary removal of the canal wall by the Wullstein [Wullstein and Wullstein, 1986] or Feldmann [1977] technique. Over the last 10 years, both these procedures have been widely accepted by supporters of closed techniques. Small cholesteatomas growing toward the epitympanum and/or the antrum are seen more often nowadays. In such cases, an atticotomy is performed by an endaural approach and the lateral attic wall is reconstructed with tragal cartilage and overlapping perichondrium [Plester, 1979].

We prefer the *open technique* with total resection of the posterior canal wall in those cases with poor pneumatization, with the sigmoid sinus far anterior, or with insufficient tubal ventilation; in elderly patients; and when adequate aftercare cannot be guaranteed. The aim is to form a small, self-cleaning cavity. The most important measures have been described by Plester [1985]. After the 'facial ridge' has been drilled down, all bony junctions and septa should be smoothed with a diamond burr. With extensive pneumatization, the bone should be drilled down to the level of the sinus and, if necessary, the mastoid tip ground down. We often reduce the size of the cavity by creating a Palva musculoperiosteal flap which is pedicled anteriorly toward the auricle; the periosteal side faces the canal.

This technique can also be used for revision surgery: even though the flap is not as well vascularized as at the primary intervention, its size remains relatively stable. One indisputable prerequisite for the execution of any obliterative measure is absolute certainty that all inflammatory foci and, especially, the entire cholesteatoma matrix can be removed.

Since 1981, after testing porous tricalcium phosphate ceramic in the middle ear of guinea pigs and rabbits (fig. 6), we have been using this material for *partial obliteration of mastoid cavities* in many revision cases. Zöllner et al. [1983] also investigated this ceramic in the mastoid of domestic pigs. Tricalcium phosphate ceramic and hydroxylapatite are bioreactive, their composition being similar to the inorganic component of bone. Given a suitable bony implant bed, porous tricalcium phosphate ceramic can be partially or totally resorbed and replaced by endogenous bony tissue, depending on the grade of porosity, the crystalline structure, and the size of the implant.

Antibiotic-impregnated ceramic serves as an antibiotic depot. After preliminary preparation of all epithelium lining the cavity, it is often advantageous to leave part of a facial ridge, if present, and to fill up the entire niche. Reliable protection of the external canal, for example, can be achieved with large grafts of autologous cartilage with overlapping perichondrium. Histologic controls showed ceramic remnants, newly formed bone, and vascular connective tissue as long as 2 years after surgery. No foreign body reactions were demonstrable. For the last 5 years, we have been using mortar-ground ceramic granulate to accelerate bony transformation in endogenous bone and to achieve more exact adaptation to the cavity or niche.

We *reconstruct the posterior canal wall* only when the defect is small enough to be covered with tragal cartilage and overlapping perichondrium (see above). Porous tricalcium phosphate ceramic is unsuitable, because the bony implant bed is inadequate and, consequently, most of the material is resorbed without bony substitution. Porous hydroxylapatite [Grote, 1984] or glass ceramic, which was introduced by the Mainz hospital, is more suitable. Given the appropriate biomechanical conditions, stable bony union can be achieved with these materials. The use of hydroxylapatite granulate together with human fibrin adhesive has also been recommended [Wullstein and Wullstein, 1986].

Even though the current trend in cholesteatoma surgery, both internationally and in our department, favors open techniques, exclusive preference of one technique over the other is to be avoided. Many patients are helped with a preserved canal wall. Our long-term hearing results were markedly better with preservation of a deep tympanic cavity [Jahnke et al., 1985]. This could partially be due to the more favorable condition of the patients with preserved posterior canal wall, e.g. less destruction of ossicular chain. Long-term controls are especially important with the closed technique. Every surgeon should create a follow-up file containing those patients for whom reoperation is indicated.

Annual controls should still be scheduled 10 years or more after surgery. The younger the patient is at the first operation, the more important are annual follow-ups. One still unanswered question is the extent to which high-resolution computerized tomography of the petrous bone will be able to replace 'second look' operations.

Surgery for Otosclerosis and Minor Malformations

Virtually no other operative method has the functional success and comparative safety of the stapedectomy. This was as true in 1970 as it is in 1987. During the last 17 years, the Plester technique (i.e. removal of the posterior part of the footplate) has been modified only insofar as, depending on the situation, no more than the posterior third, fourth, or fifth of the footplate is removed. Total removal of the stapes, which, at one time, was the procedure of choice in many hospitals, was also not done in the past, since the risk of disturbing the labyrinthine system is higher and, according to extensive comparative statistics, hearing results are not as good.

Except for the addition of a probe to determine the distance between the long process of the incus and the footplate, we have changed neither the approach nor the instruments. Fine perforations are punched in thicker footplates with a sharp trocar. For the last 7 years, we have used a platinum band Teflon prosthesis, which can be looped around the long process of the incus. The loop rarely loosens. The 4.5-mm-long standard prosthesis can be shortened with a scalpel; the diameter of the Teflon strut is 0.6 mm. The prosthesis is sealed by sheathing the Teflon component in connective tissue flaps and then folding back meticulously dissected mucosa at the border of the oval window.

In addition to long-term studies, *revision surgery* also provides valuable information on stapes surgery. An analysis of the experience gathered by many ear surgeons shows revision to be indicated in approximately 5% of all stapedectomies. We reviewed 210 patients who had undergone stapes revision surgery in the 1970s [Plester and Jahnke, 1982]. In 1986, Plester reported his experience with 1,040 stapes revisions at the Otosclerosis Symposium in Lisbon. The most frequent symptoms leading to revision were progressive hearing loss (86.4%), tinnitus (32.2%), and vertigo (8.2%). 12.4% of the revision patients with a Schuknecht wire-connective tissue prosthesis complained of dizziness. The rare failures after stapedectomy can be attributed to surgical technique-related difficulties or to the disease itself. The most frequent reasons for revision found at operation involved the prosthesis: it had migrated, was too long or too short, had loosened, or was absent. The prosthesis could not be located in 3 patients who had undergone surgery at another hospital. The wire-connective tissue stapes was frequently too short, namely, in 27% of the revision cases; the wire-Teflon prosthesis too short in 8%. Loosening of the loop around the long process of the incus (23%) could often be diagnosed on the basis of a positive tension sign, i.e. short-term hearing improvement after Valsalva's maneuver. Adhesions were an even more frequent cause of conductive deafness (36%). Loosening of the loop is frequently due to inadequate pinching of the band or erosion of the long process of the incus. Conductive deafness is pronounced when the long process is totally necrotic. A malleovestibulopexy may be necessary for chain reconstruction. The frequency of incus dislocations was 4 times higher in those patients who had initially undergone surgery in another hospital. The frequency of fistulas was also higher in these patients (5.6%), due primarily to the high number of polyethylene prostheses implanted at the other hospitals. Fistulas were found at revision in 17.4% of the cases with polyethylene prostheses, but they were extremely rare with wire-connective tissue stapes. Otospongious reclosure of the oval window was diagnosed in 15.8% of the revision patients, almost all of whom had a wire-connective tissue prosthesis. In 4 cases, a closed oval window was opened.

Particularly deserving of mention are the cases in which severe irritation of the labyrinthine system developed during the first few postoperative days. In such cases, we almost always found a foreign body granuloma caused by drape lint or talcum powder. Immediate revision is indicated in such cases which comprised 5.6% of the reoperations. The frequency of this complication has declined sharply at our hospital in the last 10 years.

Extrusion of the stapes prosthesis through the tympanic membrane is an extremely rare complication. Recently, we saw such a case; the extrusion was apparently due to a transitory impairment in ventilation and adhesion of the tympanic membrane to the long process of the incus. While the postoperative results of revision surgery were certainly an improvement over the preoperative state, they were not as good as those generally achieved at the first stapedectomy. Fortunately, bony conduction was not significantly reduced after revision. Whereas the estimated risk of deafness with primary stapedectomy is 0.5–2% (less than 0.3% in our patients), the estimated risk of deafness with stapes revision is 3–14%. This discrepancy over against our patients is best explained by the fact that we meticulously avoid opening the inner ear at revision unless bony reclosure is present. With the wire-connective tissue stapes, the wire above the knot is cut with a sharp wire cutter, the knot with connective tissue left, and the new prosthesis inserted posterior to it. This avoids tearing of the delicate walls of the endolymphatic system, which can be connected to the prosthesis by scar tissue adhesions. At the same time, the risk of infection is reduced. When, in exceptional cases, the vestibulum must be opened, a small opening for insertion of a platinum band Teflon prosthesis is created at the posterior border of the oval window niche and then sheathed with connective tissue flaps.

Stapes surgery is extremely important for *minor malformations of the ear:* an isolated stapes anomaly was present in 41% of our patients (225 minor ear malformations) and, additionally, an incus anomaly in 31%. Anomalies of the malleus and incus are frequently associated with major malformations with atretic auditory canal, but rarely with minor malformations. The tendon of the stapedius muscle was absent in 36 of 162 cases with isolated or combined stapes malformations. Due to defective development of the annular ligament, the stapes was immobile in three fourths of the patients with isolated malformation of the stapes. This group also included a pair of twins and two cousins (familial frequency, 7%). One stapes crus was deformed or a columella-shaped stapes superstructure was found in the rest of the cases. Operative treatment of isolated stapes anomalies approximates that of otosclerosis and is similarly successful. It should be noted that the distance between the long process of the incus and the footplate is often abnormally long and that the footplate should be cautiously perforated to ensure immediate recognition of a gusher phenomenon. Communication between the perilymphatic spaces and the subarachnoid space leads to an efflux of large quantities of perilymph. In such cases, the risk of deafness is relatively high. If the vestibule is already open, the best solution is the insertion of a wire-connective tissue prosthesis with a relatively large connective tissue graft. A small fenestra technique was performed successfully in one case.

If, in addition to the malformation of the stapes, the long process of the incus is also malformed, i.e. relatively delicate and vertical, a stapedectomy is not advisable in approximately one-half of the cases: the method of choice is then a malleovestibulopexy. If the oval window niche is displaced by a persisting arteria stapedia or an abnormally coursing facial nerve, the creation of a promontory window using the Plester technique has proved successful. On the basis of anatomic studies, the most favorable procedure for this operation, which is rarely indicated, has been reported by Plester and Katzke [1983]. Extensive enchondralization prevents bony closure. The prosthesis, which extends from the malleus handle approximately 0.25 mm into the perilymphatic space, is sheathed with connective tissue. Our functional results correspond well with those for stapedectomy.

Bony blocking that fixes the incus to the posteriosuperior canal wall was found in 6 of our 225 cases. After temporary disruption of the sound conduction chain, the blocking was ablated and hearing subsequently normalized.

We do not classify most cases of isolated *idiopathic fixation of the malleus head* as minor malformations, since the age distribution of the patients, the duration of their hearing impairment, and its progression tend to speak against a congenital anomaly. This, however, does not exclude the possibility that a rudimentarily narrow epitympanum may be a predisposing factor. Studies by Katzke and Plester [1981] demonstrated that, given good pneumatization, the best results are achieved by mobilization of the malleus head, obviously with temporary chain disruption. As experience with more than 300 cases has shown, this procedure is not recommended for cases with poor pneumatization. In such cases, the method with the most favorable results at present is removal of the incus and malleus head, followed by ossicle interposition. Time will tell whether further improvements will be achieved by removing excess bone or part of the malleus head with a laser.

In conclusion, it should be noted that one important advancement in middle ear surgery is the reduction of the complication rate. According to Miehlke, in the 1970s, the facial nerve was injured during surgery in almost 1% of all interventions on the middle ear and, according to the literature, in 4.6–11% of the revision cases. The drastic reduction of these high complication rates is unquestionably due to the improved training of ear surgeons. Residents in Tübingen are required to perform 22 different operations on cadaveric petrous bones before they are allowed to perform their first ear operation; the quality of surgery is controlled under the operating microscope by Prof. Plester. The training in microsurgery of the ear, which ultimately leads to improved operative results, is provided by regular seminars, 20 of which have been held to date in Tübingen.

In summary, many advancements have been made in middle ear surgery during the last 15 years. Even though no truly new concepts have been introduced, these advances have been made possible by many technical refinements. Given correct establishment of the indication, these refinements have made possible an extremely differentiated and individually tailored microsurgery.

References

Cousins, V.; Jahnke, K.: Light and electronmicroscopic studies on Polycel™ ossicular replacement prostheses. Clin. Otolaryngol. *12:* 183–189 (1987).

Feldmann, H.: Osteoplastische Meato-Attiko-Antrotomie. Lar. Rhinol. Otol. *56:* 786–795 (1977).

Frootko, N.: Causes of ossiculoplasty failure using porous polyethylene (Plastipore) prostheses; in Grote, Biomaterials in otology, pp. 169–171 (Nijhoff, Boston 1984).

Gerlach, H.: Die Stepp-Plastik zur Erhaltung der Trommelfellebene. Arch. Ohr.-Nas.-KehlkHeilk. *202:* 662–665 (1972).

Grote, J.J.: Biomaterials in otology, pp. 274–280 (Nijhoff, Boston 1984).

Heermann, H.; Heermann, J.: Endaurale Chirurgie (Urban & Schwarzenberg, München 1964).

Helms, J.: Die Wiederherstellung der Schalleitungskette. HNO *31:* 37–44 (1983).

Jahnke, K.; Khatib, M.; Rau, U.: Langzeitergebnisse nach Cholesteatomchirurgie. Lar. Rhinol. Otol. *64:* 238–242 (1985).

Jahnke, K.; Plester, D.: Keramik-Implantate in der Mittelohrchirurgie. HNO *28:* 109–114 (1980a).

Jahnke, K.; Plester, D.: Praktische Hinweise zur Anwendung von Mittelohrimplantaten aus Aluminiumoxid-Keramik. HNO *28:* 115–118 (1980b).

Jahnke, K.; Schrader, M.: Kohlenstoffimplantate im Mittelohr. Archs Oto-Rhino-Lar., suppl. II, pp. 52–54 (1984).

Jahnke, K.; Strohm, M.: Zur Chirurgie der kleinen Ohrmissbildungen. 64. Versammlung südwestdeutscher HNO-Ärzte, Bad Kissingen 1980.

Katzke, D.; Plester, D.: Idiopathic malleus head fixation as a cause of a combined conductive and sensorineural hearing loss. Clin. Otolaryngol. 6: 39–44 (1981).

Kerr, A.G.: Proplast and Plastipore. Clin. Otolaryngol. 6: 187–191 (1981).

Kley, W.: Operative Behandlung der chronischen Otitis media und ihrer unmittelbaren Folgezustände; in Naumann, Kopf- und Halschirurgie, vol. 3 (Thieme, Stuttgart 1976).

Merwin, M.D.: Bioglass middle ear prothesis. Preliminary report. Ann. Otol. Rhinol. Lar. 95: 78–82 (1986).

Plester, D.: Fortschritte in der Mikrochirurgie des Ohres in den letzten 10 Jahren. HNO 18: 33–40 (1970).

Plester, D.: Chirurgie des Cholesteatoms. Archs Oto-Rhino-Lar. 223: 380–390 (1979).

Plester, D.: Mastoidchirurgie früher und heute. 68. Versammlung südwestdeutscher HNO-Ärzte, Bad Homburg 1985.

Plester, D.; Jahnke, K.: Erfahrungen bei Stapesnachoperationen. 66. Versammlung südwestdeutscher HNO-Ärzte, Ulm 1982.

Plester, D.; Katzke, D.: The promontorial window technique. Laryngoscope 83: 824–825 (1983).

Plester, D.; Pusalkar, A.: The anterior tympanomeatal angle. The aetiology, surgery and avoidance of blunting and annular cholesteatoma. Clin. Otolaryngol. 6: 323–328 (1981).

Plester, D.; Zöllner, F.: Behandlung der chronischen Mittelohrentzündungen; in Berendes, Link, Zöllner, Hals-Nasen-Ohrenheilkunde in Praxis und Klinik; 2. Aufl., vol. 6, p. 28 (Thieme, Stuttgart 1980).

Reck, R.: 5 Jahre klinische Erfahrungen mit Ceravitalprothesen im Mittelohr. HNO 33: 166–170 (1985).

Shea, J.J.; Emmett, J.R.; Smyth, G.D.L.: Biocompatible implants in otology. ORL 39: 9–15 (1977).

Shea, J.J.; Moretz, W.H.: Peg tip fixation on Plastipore-TORP. Otolar. HN Surg. 93: 279–280 (1984).

Smyth, G.D.L.; Kerr, A.G.: Homologous grafts for ossicular reconstruction in tympanoplasty. Laryngoscope, St. Louis 77: 330–336 (1967).

Steinbach, E.; Pusalkar, A.: Long-term histological fate of cartilage in ossicular reconstruction. J. Lar. Otol. 95: 1031–1039 (1981).

Utech, H.: Bessere Endhörergebnisse bei Tympanoplastik durch Veränderung der Operationstechnik. Z. Lar. Rhinol. Otol. 39: 367–371 (1960).

Wullstein, H.L.; Wullstein, S.R.: Tympanoplastik: Osteoplastische Epitympanotomie (Thieme, Stuttgart 1986).

Zöllner, C.; Strutz, J.; Beck, Chl.; Büsing, C.M.; Jahnke, K.; Heimke, G.: Verödung des Warzenfortsatzes mit poröser Trikalzium-Phosphat-Keramik. Lar. Rhinol. 62: 106–111 (1983).

Zöllner, F.: Tympanosclerosis. Archs Otolar. 78: 538–544 (1963).

Prof. Dr. Klaus Jahnke, Universitäts-HNO-Klinik, Feulgenstrasse 10, D–6300 Giessen (FRG)

Adv. Oto-Rhino-Laryng., vol. 39, pp. 83–93 (Karger, Basel 1988)

Modern Surgical Concepts in the Treatment of Chronic Middle Ear Disease[1]

C. Deguine

Lille, France

We are all aware of the significant progress in the realm of surgery for chronic otitis which has been made in recent years [1, 11]. These acquisitions, both in theory and in practice, have permitted us to increase the reliability and safety of our procedures, as well as to augment the scope of our indications for surgery.

It is above all comforting to realize that these interventions, once questioned by our patients, have gained their confidence. They come now not only for a remedy for a draining ear, but more and more often asking for a surgical solution for simple hearing loss.

The reputation of surgery for deafness has grown equally in the eyes of our colleagues. More and more of our young interns are seeking places in our training programs, quite the opposite of the situation in the not too distant past.

Noteworthy progress in another area needs to be mentioned. These are the extraordinary possibilities for teaching and communication offered by our modern audiovisual systems. Microsurgery used to be a rather private affair when the neophytes had to share an inverted lateral observer tube. Those who knew that era cannot help but admire video, which affords the observer a color image as good if not better than that of the surgeon, along with a sound track and the capability to record, view and comment on at one's leisure.

However, the task of the young otologist is complicated by the variety of principles, techniques and materials used, from which he must now choose. If concepts on certain points are different, or even radically opposed, it may be because many department chiefs feel the need to teach

[1] I wish to thank Dr. Lee Miller, Shape Hospital, Mons (Belgium), for his guidance in the preparation and translation of the paper.

one well-established, often simplified method, that can be easily dupli-
cated in the majority of cases. This does not always dovetail with the variety of pathology and the situations which must be handled. If the rule
dictates that the best is the simplest, it does not always hold true that the
simplest is the best. In reality nothing is really simple.

It is in this view that we propose a discussion of modern trends in the
surgery of chronic middle ear disease focusing on three essential chapters:
myringoplasty; ossiculoplasty; cholesteatoma.

Myringoplasty

The choice of grafting materials is not the critical problem. The attributes of temporalis fascia – availability, accessibility, ease of handling and
high degree of take, are evident in view of its widespread utilization. Some
recommend tragal perichondrium as the material of first choice, because of
its more rigid structure, which would tend to reduce the risk of retraction.
Other materials can be used with some degree of success. According to the
circumstances (revision surgery, transcanal approach, or others), vein, periosteum, homografts of fascia, dura, heart valves or heterograft calf veins
(Neotymp) may be appropriate.

In the past 15 years great interest in tympanic homografts had developed through the work of Marquet [10]. At the present time only a small
number of surgeons continue to utilize this method as their prefered technique. The principal reasons for this loss of interest reside in cost, problems in obtaining the tissue and a degree of take which is lower than that of
autogenous material. Tympanic homografts still find an indication in certain functional problems, or in the delicate treatment of agenesis.

The controversial point in the utilization of the connective tissue graft
is in the technique of application: overlay or underlay.

The most frequently seen complications of myringoplasty are: residual
pearls, blunting of the anterior sulcus, and lateralization of the graft.

The underlay technique, in which the graft is applied to the undersur-
face of the drum remnant, avoids these 3 risks. It thus offers a certain
advantage, especially for the young surgeon. It is indicated in all cases
where it appears feasible.

As simple as it may appear, several difficulties arise in regard to main-
taining it in position. Filling the middle ear with absorbable gelatin sponge
(gelfoam) is contrary to our philosophy of keeping this space as well ven-

tilated as possible. Its fixation by natural adherence or surface tension is adequate only for small perforations. The use of biologic glue has been disappointing in our experience. Creating small button-holes in the drum remnants, according to the technique of Gerlach, is an effective means of stabilization. However, we have observed delays in healing and cases of postoperative myringitis. The most commonly used method consists of elevating the fibrous annulus and applying the graft to the bony canal. We will see later the considerations which lead us to respect this anatomic structure as much as possible.

The so-called simple myringoplasty represents only a limited fraction in the surgery of chronic middle ear disease. Apart from cholesteatoma, in about one-half of the cases, there exists an associated ossicular problem and the application of an underlay graft could compromise the adjustment of the columella in its contact with the handle of the malleus.

Finally, there are a significant number of myringoplasties where it becomes necessary to meticulously separate the epithelium which has migrated toward the middle ear, as in the case of a retraction pocket or an 'epidermosis': these are the atelectasic ear, the so-called pre-cholesteatomas. If the surgeon is capable of identifying, dissecting and accomplishing a complete removal of all epithelial remnants in this situation, the preparation of the bed of the graft for an overlay technique is possible.

The overlay technique certainly appears to be more delicate, but it offers advantages [4]. The stability of the graft is better controlled. Its use necessitates taking great care to avoid the aforementioned complications.

Prevention of the Epidermal Inclusion Cyst

A meticulous surgical technique must be used. When the epithelium has been dissected, the suction tip should be of just sufficient calibre to raise the tissue without tearing it. Keeping it intact guarantees complete removal. Reapplied to the graft, it helps to hold it in position, brings nutrition and adds to its ultimate epithelialization.

At the free edge of a perforation, the site of the mucocutaneous separation is variable. Removal of a small peripheral ring of tissue (so-called 'safety-rim') increases the size of one perforation but decreases the risk of inclusion cysts.

Long-term otomicroscopic follow-up is required in each case: yearly examination for at least 5 years. In a series of 155 cases operated on in 1975 using the overlay technique and followed over a period of 10 years, the incidence of epidermal inclusion was 4%.

Prevention of Lateralization

The normal tympanic membrane has a conical shape. To restore this with a flat piece of tissue is a challenge. In effect, experience shows that grafted temporalis fascia has a natural tendency to return to its original shape, in spite of the fact that it has been dried and moulded. A graft applied to the outer surface or the drum remnant is subject to a movement of external migration or lateralization, which separates it from the handle of the malleus. It loses its role as a vibrating membrane, to become a veritable obstacle to the passage of sound vibrations (fig. 1).

A logical method to prevent this occurrence consists of placing the graft under the handle of the malleus. We have observed that even though the incidence of lateral migration is reduced, it is not prevented. For this reason, we preserve the drum remnant, even plaques of tympanosclerosis, in order to create an even greater surface opposing the tendency for external migration (fig. 2).

Prevention of Blunting of the Anterior Angle

The anterior wall of the external auditory canal forms a very acute angle with the tympanic membrane. If a temporalis fascia graft is applied to the drum remnant, and, reflected on the anterior bony wall, if it is thick and ultimately thickened by oedema, the chances are good that blunting will occur. Moreover, because of the frequent anterior canal wall bulge, the approach to this region is delicate. Three rules must be adhered to to prevent blunting of the anterior angle.

(1) Respect of canal skin: Some recommend drilling of the bony canal. They remove and replace the canal skin as a free graft or create a large flap (while others decorate their burrs with it ...). Proceeding with the principle that tissues which have not been incised heal the best, our attitude is conservative. It can be shown, that with a correct angle of view, access to the region of the anterior drum is possible and of satisfactory degree. The only exceptions are in congenital malformations or in the presence of exostosis. If the obstacle is due to the retractors or soft tissue, the position of the soft tissue can be changed and the retractors adjusted. Finally, drilling Henle's spine or the cribiform area may prove useful. The skin of the canal should be lifted carefully, avoiding any tear. This stage may appear delicate but does not present any insurmountable difficulty, provided that one has: (a) a bloodless field permitting the use of tiny suction tubes to hold the skin flap without tearing, and (b) instruments with proper bend to avoid trauma to the skin over the anterior wall bulge.

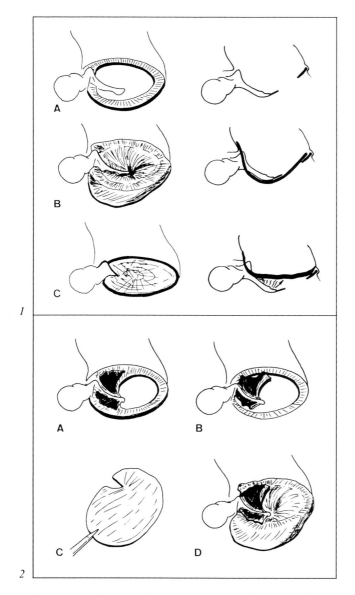

Fig. 1. Lateralization of tympanic graft. *A* Central perforation. *B* Graft applied under the malleus handle. *C* However, lateralization may occur after several years.

Fig. 2. Personal technique of tympanic membrane grafting. *A* Central perforation with plaques of tympanoclerosis. *B* Preparation of the bed of the graft. *C* Dried fascia graft with a notch. *D* Application of the graft under the malleus handle and the tympanic remnants and over the annulus.

(2) Respect of the fibrous annulus: Preservation of the fibrous annulus seems to be an important factor for the following reasons: (a) It delimits the boundary between the middle and external ear; that is, the exact position of the tympanic membrane. (b) It offers a point of support which is necessary and sufficient to fix the graft, without reflecting it over the anterior wall. (c) It is the site of an annular vascular network, mainly from the anterior tympanic artery. (d) Its assumed role in the embryogenesis of the lamina propria of the drum should instinctively engender our respect.

(3) Precise placement of the graft: The anterior edge on the graft must be applied precisely on the annulus, so as to avoid its extension to the anterior bony canal wall.

Plester and Pusalkar [13] have shown, based on systematic histological studies of temporal bones, the possibility of papillary epithelial invaginations. We have not observed any particular incidence of annular cholesteatoma, perhaps due to the meticulous technique used.

Ossiculoplasty

Apart from Wullstein type IV and V tympanoplasties, which are never better performed than by nature itself, the trend is to restore the columnellar effect. A great variety of procedures have been described, and familiarity with these is useful. One may be confronted with a multiplicity of situations, and so no single technique is universally recognized or necessarily more advantageous. Nevertheless, some general principles and tendencies merit our consideration.

Regarding material, human tissue, autogenous bone and cartilage or homografts have proved their reliability over the years.

Ossicular transposition, which we prefer [3], is exposed to resorption and above all to bony fixation to the Fallopian canal, promontory or bony annulus (fig. 3).

Cartilage does not undergo fixation. On the other hand, its use is technically more delicate. Tragal cartilage in a child or in a female is less solid than in the male. Steinbach and Pusalkar [15] have shown the risk of long-term alteration as well.

The chronically infected ear is intolerant to metal and plastic, either solid or porous [6].

Ceramics, with a chemical structure close to that of bone, offer a promising alternative. It is to the German School, and primarily to Prof.

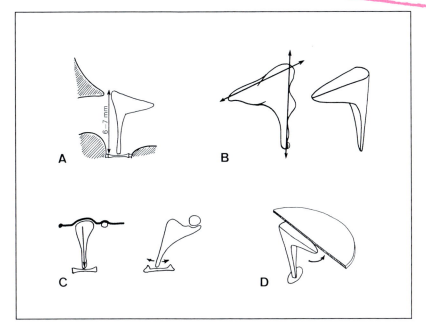

Fig. 3. Incus homograft transposition on the stapes footplate. *A* The intact incus has been found to present the exact size, tympanic ring to footplate. *B* The short process is sculpted to contact the vibrating membrane, the long process is sculpted to fit the oval window niche. *C* Its position, perpendicular to the footplate decreases risk of sleeping. *D* Pressure on the footplate may be adjusted by moving or rotating the ossicle under the slanted surface.

Plester, that we owe their introduction. They are inorganic crystalline materials, endowed with three essential biologic properties: biocompatibility, biodegradability and bioactivity. There are a certain number of these at our disposal and we will mention the two most commonly used: Frialit® [8, 9], highly purified aluminium oxide (A12 O3) which is bioinert (Plester, Jahnke) and Ceravital® [7], which is a bioactive material (Helms, Reck).

The applicability of these materials depends upon the practical experience of the surgeon. It is a pity to note in the literature of ossicular chain reconstruction, such a preponderance in the number of papers pertaining to biocompatibility and the clinical results, and such penury in regard to fundamental work on the physiology of the columella. Thus, the presence of a malleus handle in a drum remnant constitutes a favorable situation of which we should take advantage either (1) to better capture sound energy transmitted by the vibratory membrane – our observation is that the most effective assemblies are those which establish a bridge between the malleus handle and the head or footplate of the stapes, (2) to stabilize a columella; the position of the stapes or of the oval window niche in relation to the handle of the malleus is variable (a longer distance makes a direct connection precarious, but a columella applied directly under the drum can prove efficient, the handle is thus an additional stabilizing element).

Surgery for Cholesteatoma

Cholesteatoma is the most serious form of chronic otitis, because it is evolutional, engenders destructive processes and potentiates complications. Its management is in essence more delicate, because cholesteatoma in reality is the manifestation of a condition. Even if surgery preserves anatomy and restores auditory function, if the etiologic factors themselves persist, the disease process may return with retraction, recurrence or ventilatory problems.

For the past 20 years the merits of the open versus closed techniques have been debated.

The closed technique theorically represents the most satisfactory solution, since it strives to preserve near normal middle ear anatomy. In reality, the price has been a certain percentage of failure, which naturally leads to an open technique... we would like to briefly discuss our results with the closed technique [3].

Residual cholesteatoma is controlled by staged intervention with the revision scheduled about a year after the first procedure. It would be wrong if not malicious to confuse its incidence with failure since a second look permits almost total security.

The retraction pocket on the contrary constitutes a case of true failure, which justifies for certain authors the limits for the indications of this technique:

(1) Its incidence escapes our ability to prevent it: it has been reduced significantly but not eliminated by routine reconstruction of the lateral attic wall.

(2) It can appear in the long term. We have seen it occur 10 years after an apparent cure.

(3) It is difficult to predict.

The open technique eliminates by definition the risk of a retraction pocket. However, it makes possible a new type of pathology: the cavity being more or less a problem, depending on its size and shape. The current trend is to cover the walls of the mastoid cavity with connective tissue. In such a manner, the cells which were impossible to eliminate totally are obliterated, and nutritional substrate is available for epithelialization. At the very minimum this covering is constituted by fascia. It can go as far as total obliteration, with free auto-transplanted tissue or pedicled flap (Palva), periosteum or bone pâté, to partial obliteration, in the attempt to create a self-cleaning cavity.

An intermediate technique consists of enlarging the atticotomy from within to be reconstructed by: (a) a bone flap (epitympanotomy of Wullstein [16] or the osteotomy of Feldman [5]), or (b) tragal cartilage and perichondrium (Plester).

Without desiring to enter into polemics which will be with us for some years to come, it seems of interest to note that a consensus is forming for certain indications: (a) in a sclerotic mastoid, as in older patients, most authors prefer the creation of a small cavity, and (b) in the presence of a widely pneumatized mastoid, frequent in children, many prefer leaving the posterior canal wall intact. Between these extremes, attitudes vary, taking into consideration the functionality of the patient, his necessities and reliability, and of the operator, his personal experience and competence.

Miscellaneous: Tissue Glue

The surgery in chronic ear disease is overall reconstructive surgery, with the superposition of mobile and separate elements. The introduction of tissue glue would have to be a priori of great advantage (excluding the risk of transmission of modern diseases related to the use of blood by-products).

There is an unavoidable principle in plastic surgery: all transplanted material has to fit with a spontaneous and natural stability. Overcorrections, tensions, artificially induced tractions may ultimately lead to shifting. Egyptians built the pyramids without cement. That may be the reason why are they so nicely preserved! Tissue glue has to be considered as a passive element of security, rather than an active tool of middle ear repair. Neophytes who would consider it as a God send to cover their technical inexperience risk being disappointed.

However, tissue glue may be of great help to solve particular problems. In our opinion, it can give more security when used in a timely manner but should not be depended on by itself to ensure the stability of a reconstruction. The net prevents the trapeze artist from fatal accident, but does not tie him to the trapeze!

Conclusions

In closing, we would like to mention our problem child and scape goat, the Eustachian tube, whose role has been differently interpreted. It is worthy to note that the treatment of chronic middle ear disease began 2 centuries ago, with its catheterization (Itard's probe). It is only much later that we were able to see the drum in the darkness of the external ear canal. We really have not progressed much in the treatment of its dysfunction – even regressed if we consider the rarity of Eustachian tube procedures today.

We are grateful to it for having provided an excuse for our failures. However, our results have improved considerably. Sheehy has even suggested that tympanoplasty is the treatment of tubal dysfunction. It remains at the center of our preoccupations. The key to the problem lies probably in a better understanding of the physiology and physiopathology of the tubo-tympanic mucosa. There still remains a great deal of work for future generations of otologists.

References

1   Austin, D.F.: A decade of tympanoplasty. Progress or regress? Larnygoscope 92: 527–530 (1982).
2   Deguine, C.: Le traitement chirurgical du cholestéatome en technique fermée. Annls Otolar. 97: 99–103 (1980).
3   Deguine, C.: Tympanoplastie: restauration fonctionnelle en cas de lyse des branches de l'étrier. J. fr. ORL 31–10: 737–744 (1982).
4   Deguine, C.: La réparation de la membrane tympanique. Sté Franç. d'ORL et de Pathol. cervico-faciale. C.r. séanc. Libr. Arnette 1984: 450–454.
5   Feldmann, H.: Surgeon's workshop: osteoplastic approach in chronic otitis media by means of a microsurgical reciprocating saw. Clin. Otolar. 3: 515–520 (1978).
6   Frootko, N.J.: Failed ossiculoplasty using porous polyethylene (plasti-pore) prostheses. 1st Int. Symp. Univ. Leiden, the Netherlands Politzer Society 1983: 29.
7   Helms, J.: Reconstruction of the ossicular chain; in Marquet, Surgery and pathology of the middle ear, pp. 113–116 (1984).

8   Heumann, H.; Jahnke, K.; Plester, D.: La tolérance d'une céramique à l'oxyde d'aluminium dans la chirurgie de l'oreille moyenne. Sté Franç. d'ORL et de Pathol. cervico-faciale. C.r. séanc. Libr. Arnette *1979:* 89–91.

9   Jahnke, K.; Plester, D.: Bioinert ceramic implants in middle ear surgery. Ann. Otolar. *90:* 640–642 (1981).

10 Marquet, J.: Ten years of experience in tympanoplasty using homologous implants. J. Lar. Otol. *10:* 897–905 (1976).

11 Plester, D.: Fortschritte in der Mikrochirurgie des Ohres in den letzten 10 Jahren. HNO *18:* 33–40 (1970).

12 Plester, D.: Short- and long-term results in ossiculoplasty in cholesteatomatous ears. Cholesteatoma and mastoid surgery. Proc. IInd Int. Conf., Tel Aviv, Israel 1981, p. 571 (Kugler, Amsterdam 1982).

13 Plester, D.; Pusalkar, A.: The anterior tympanomeatal angle: the aetiology, surgery and avoidance of blunting and annular cholesteatoma. Clin. otolar. *6:* 323–328 (1981).

14 Reck, R.; Helms, J.: The bioactive glass ceramic ceravital in ear surgery. Five years' experience. Am. J. Otol. *6:* 280–283 (1985).

15 Steinbach, E.; Pusalkar, A.: Long-term histological fate of cartilage in ossicular reconstruction. J. Lar. Otol. *95:* 1031–1309 (1981).

16 Wullstein, H.L.; Wullstein, S.R.: Tympanoplastik. Osteoplastische Epitympanotomie (Thieme, Stuttgart 1986).

Dr. C. Deguine, 134, bd de la Liberté, F–59800 Lille (France)

Adv. Oto-Rhino-Laryng., vol. 39, pp. 94–106 (Karger, Basel 1988)

Cholesteatoma – Pathology and Treatment

E. Steinbach[a], *A. Pusalkar*[b], *H. Heumann*[a]

[a] Department of Otorhinolaryngology, University of Tübingen, Tübingen, FRG;
[b] Department of Otolaryngology, TN Medical College and BYL Nair Hospital, Bombay, India

Introduction

The pathology of cholesteatoma can be simply defined as invasion of the middle ear space by squamous epithelium from the external auditory canal. What is the reason for so much interest in inflammation in this small area? Why in the last 10 years have two international conferences been devoted to this problem? There are many reasons. We are all aware that chronic inflammation of the middle ear mucosa, tympanosclerosis, cholesterol granuloma, etc. behave differently from cholesteatoma. Complications are rare in cases of tympanosclerosis and almost never occur in tubotympanic catarrh. Cholesteatoma, on the other hand, behaves in an entirely different way. It frequently leads to partial or total destruction of ossicles but, surprisingly perhaps, the footplate is always spared. In addition, it often causes facial paralysis and may be the source of intracranial infection. It is a remarkable phenomenon that the same epithelium which protects the ear canal can cause extensive destruction in the middle ear. Until today, no satisfactory explanation has been put forward for the peculiar behaviour of cholesteatoma.

Many reports have suggested that destruction takes place only when the cholesteatoma is secondarily infected. In reality, however, bone destruction is seen even in the absence of infection. Similarly, earlier theories which suggested that pressure was a cause of bone destruction only hold true in a small percentage of cases. These theories say that the pressure of the keratin in the cholesteatoma sac leads to pressure necrosis of the surrounding bone. It can be shown in experimental animals that cholesteatoma causes bone destruction even when it has adequate space. Many authors have suggested that stratified squamous epithelium is not the cause of bone destruction because squamous epithelium itself is never actually in direct contact with bone. The epithelium causes only progressive osteitis.

The function of the Eustachian tube seems to be the most important contributing factor. From our own clinical observations, we feel that the progression of cholesteatoma may be due to minor dysfunction of the Eustachian tube causing gradually inadequate aeration of the middle ear cleft. In contrast, the rapid onset of complete obstruction of the tube causes a mucotympanum.

Animal Experiments

Several animal experiments are in progress in the Department of ORL of the University of Tübingen to investigate the aetiology of cholesteatoma formation. In addition, many biopsies taken from the middle ear during surgery are being examined. The questions being investigated are: Is there a preferred site for cholesteatoma formation and, if so, why? Is an irritant factor necessary and, if so, at which particular site? Is the irritant factor necessary in the external auditory canal or in the middle ear? What about the Eustachian tube?

With these questions in mind, the experiments were divided into three main groups. In the first group (experiments 1–3) we used mild irritants to produce inflammation at different sites lateral to the tympanic membrane. In the second group (4 and 5) inflammation was induced directly in the middle ear without disturbing the tympanic membrane. Finally, in experiment 6 the Eustachian tube was closed (fig. 1).

Animal Experiment 1

Irritants were placed in the antero-inferior typanomeatal angle and left in situ for up to 6 months. The irritants used were gelfoam, histoacrylate tissue glue and talcum. Surprisingly, though inflammation of the tympanic membrane was seen, in no case there was any inflammation specifically in the postero-superior area or cholesteatoma formation.

Animal Experiment 2

Irritants (histoacrylic tissue glue and gelfoam) were placed directly on the postero-superior segment. Eighty-six percent of these animals showed the typical formation of cholesteatoma with infiltrating squamous epithelium, cholesteatoma matrix and a keratin-filled sac, and also rarefying osteitis.

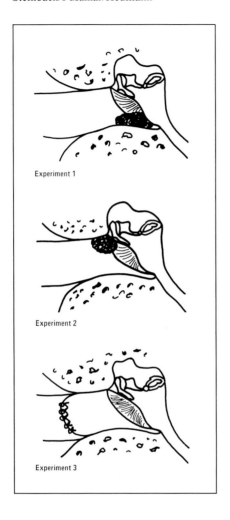

Experiment 1

Experiment 2

Experiment 3

Fig. 1. Animal experiments 1–6.

Animal Experiments 3

The external auditory canal was closed with sutures creating a blind sac. After four weeks, severe inflammation was seen in this sac, with hyperaemia and an inflammatory cell infiltrate. The composition of this material resembled a cholesteatoma sac, and this inflammation caused destruction specifically of the pars flaccida with the formation of cholesteatoma. Interestingly, ingrowth of squamous epithelium was not seen in the antero-inferior quadrant of the tympanic membrane, though there was inflammation in this area.

Animal Experiment 4

In this group, gelfoam and histoacrylate were placed directly in the middle ear of the rabbits by opening the bulla laterally without disturbing the tympanic membrane. The irritants were placed, with the help of a small laryngeal mirror, on the long process of the incus, the handle of malleus and the medial aspect of the tympanic membrane. There was a severe inflammatory reaction around the ossicles and in the middle ear cleft, but in no case there was formation of cholesteatoma.

Animal Experiment 5

Grafting of a piece of bone with overlying epidermis by a lateral approach. A piece of bone of the size of the incus was removed from the external auditory meatus and placed with its overlying skin in the middle ear. After 8 weeks, the skin had developed into a classical cholesteatoma. The piece of implanted bone showed lacuna formation but there was little inflammatory reaction. At the site of removal of this bone, the skin showed ingrowths of epithelium in the canal with the characteristics of a canal cholesteatoma. This was also a progressive cholesteatoma.

Animal Experiment 6

A tympanomeatal flap was raised and the Eustachian tube orifice was closed with muscle. Cholesteatoma formation was observed in the region of the pars flaccida.

Conclusions from These Experiments

(1) When cholesteatoma was observed, it always appeared at a specific place, the postero-superior segment. This area corresponds to the pars flaccida in humans. The predilection of cholesteatoma for this area is perhaps due to the particular anatomical structure of the pars flaccida. Histologically, this region has a varying thickness of connective tissue rich in blood vessels. Inflammation of the pars flaccida is characterised by an increase in the subepithelial connective tissue with increased vascularity. Inflammation allows the squamous epithelium to grow into the deeper connective tissue layer towards the epitympanic recess and middle ear. Due to this ingrowth, the cells of the stratum germinatum change their growth axis with a vertical penetration of the basal layer. The epithelial cones start keratinising and accumulate debris in the centre, thus forming a typical

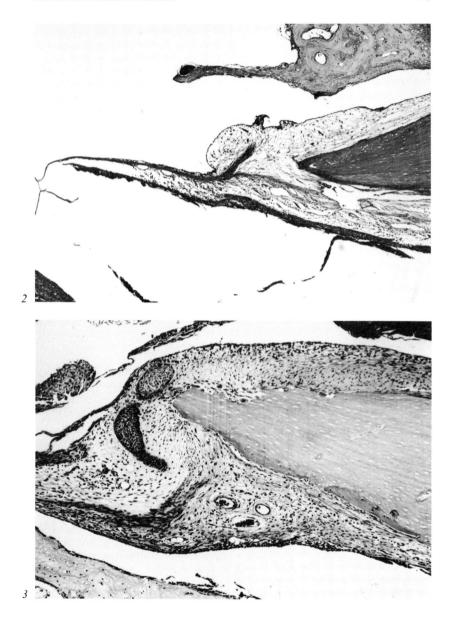

Fig. 2. Thickening of the epidermis of the pars flaccida 2 weeks after irritation of that area with histoacrylate. HE. × 40.

Fig. 3. Two weeks later a few epithelial cones were seen in the submucous connective tissue. HE. × 100.

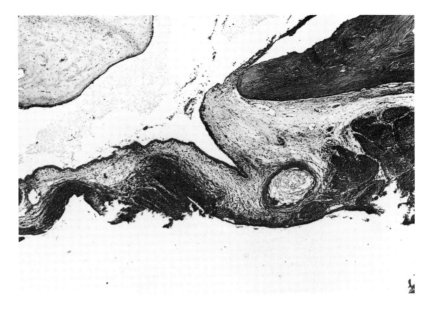

Fig. 4. In other animals the development of small epidermis cysts is observed. HE.
× 80.

cholesteatoma. The remarkable feature of cholesteatoma is that the irritating factor must be lateral to the tympanic membrane. Irritants in the middle ear did not produce a cholesteatoma (fig. 2–7).

(2) The progression of cholesteatoma was not always accompanied by bacterial infection; in many experiments there was a dry cholesteatoma with rarefying osteitis.

(3) Experiment 5 showed that bone destruction is not due to pressure necrosis. The classical hypothesis that the squamous epithelial matrix is filled with debris causes pressure on the bone leading to necrosis does not hold true. The detailed examination of the cellular pattern in cholesteatoma in many animal experiments showed loose connective tissue with dense cells lying between the cholesteatoma matrix and neighbouring bone. The cells most frequently observed were fibroblasts, lymphocytes, plasma cells and eosinophilic granulocytes. The presence of these types of cells suggests that rarefying osteitis is caused by an enzymatic process [Abramson et al., 1975].

On the basis of recent immunological studies, Gantz [1984] has put forward his own hypothesis for rarefying osteitis in cholesteatoma. He

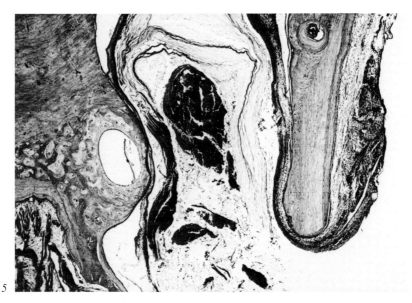

5

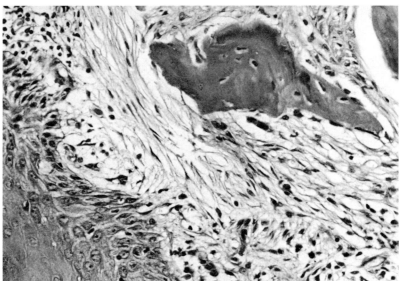

6

Fig. 5. After 8 weeks the presence of cholesteatoma in the epitympanon is found. HE. × 80.

Fig. 6. The lateral wall of the epitympanon is partly destroyed by cholesteatoma matrix. HE. × 300.

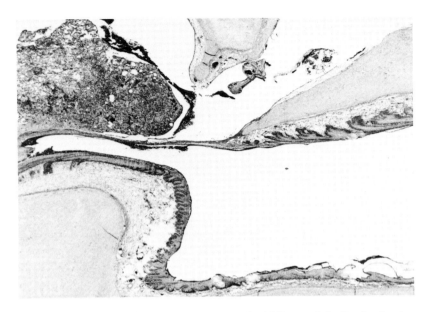

Fig. 7. There is no reaction at the eardrum and middle ear cleft after implanting gelfoam by a lateral approach. HE. $\times$ 40.

suggested that the epidermal Langerhans' cells in the cholesteatoma sac become sensitised to non-specific antigens. These cells' activated lymphocytes wander to the irritated part causing an inflammatory reaction followed by bone erosion.

Histological Findings in Granulating Myringitis

As previously mentioned, histological slides of biopsies from human middle ears and tympanic membranes were also studied. Interesting pathology was noted in granular myringitis. According to Schuknecht [1974], the squamous epithelium of the tympanic membrane is replaced by a thin layer of granulation tissue. The 23 tympanic membrane biopsies we examined showed histological findings surprisingly similar to those seen in the early development of cholesteatoma. In very inflamed tissue, an unusually marked ingrowth of epithelial cones was noticeable. This squamous epithelium reached near to the middle ear mucosa and was surrounded by a dense capillary network with a round cell infiltrate. From these histological findings, we think that granular myringitis may be a precursor of cholesteatoma.

Summary

(1) The prerequisite for development of cholesteatoma is a cholesteatoma bed, that is a loose subepithelial connective tissue layer which acts as a nutrient bed and makes papillary growth of squamous epithelium possible.

(2) The formation of cholesteatoma is facilitated by disturbed tubal function with reduced ventilation of the middle ear.

(3) The progression of cholesteatoma, especially the bone destruction, is due to enzyme-activated cell groups.

The epidermal layer in the postero-superior area of the tympanic membrane has a higher papillary content and during an inflammatory process there is a marked vascular reaction. This particular area has a special nutritional zone and the epidermis is especially well nourished [Lange, 1925]. The main artery to the tympanic membrane travels along the handle of the malleus and gives off branches. In our animal experiments epithelial cones grew into this well-nourished subepithelial zone and formed cholesteatoma.

The importance of tubal function as regards cholesteatoma formation can be seen in everyday clinical practice. In stapedectomy patients, the lateral attic wall is usually removed to allow full visualisation of the stapes, but retraction pockets in this area are never seen at subsequent follow-up. However, if the lateral attic wall is removed during surgery for chronic otitis media, reconstruction with cartilage or ceramic is necessary to prevent retraction. This adds weight to the hypothesis that tubal dysfunction is an important aetiological factor in cholesteatoma. This is further supported by the 30 times greater incidence of retraction pockets in patients with cleft palate.

Management of Cholesteatoma

As far as management is concerned, the aetiology of a cholesteatoma, be it primary, secondary or traumatic, is of secondary importance. Removal of squamous epithelium from the middle ear is the only successful treatment. Conservative measures, such as topical medication or suction clearance, are of purely temporary benefit. There is a considerable difference between the treatment of attico-antral and tubo-tympanic disease. A discharging ear in tubo-tympanic disease can usually be controlled by local toilet and topical or systemic medication. Occasionally, even spontaneous closure of a perforation occurs. The spontaneous disappearance of a cholesteatoma is never seen. The management of a cholesteatoma is surgical. The primary aim of surgery is removal of the cholesteatoma matrix from the middle ear cleft. The secondary aim should be preservation or improvement of the hearing. As advocated by Plester [1979], patients with cholesteatoma are treated by one of three methods: (1) posterior tympano-tomy (combined approach tympanoplasty); (2) atticotomy with recon-struction of the lateral attic wall; (3) attico-antrostomy or modified radical mastoidectomy.

Posterior Tympanotomy

It is an exciting idea to eliminate the cholesteatoma by the combina-tion of an anterior and posterior approach and to achieve not only removal of the pathological process but also preservation of a large middle ear volume and the physiological self-cleaning capacity of the external ear. An important prerequisite for this procedure is an average or well-pneuma-tized mastoid. The advantage of this technique is the preservation of the posterior canal wall. When the extent of the cholesteatoma is determined, either from pre-operative X-rays or clinically by passing a probe into the retraction pocket, the type of operation can be decided. The details of the operation are not discussed here.

Good pneumatisation is essential. Cholesteatoma often gets deeply embedded in the mastoid air cells. After removal of the matrix and peri-matrix, the neighbouring bone area must be carefully drilled in order to be certain that the squamous epithelial remnants are completely removed.

The advantage of this procedure is that the bony external auditory canal remains anatomically unaltered, but there are definite disadvan-tages. Firstly, the site of origin of the cholesteatoma and its spread into the sinus tympani cannot be visualised under the operating microscope through this approach. Some parts of the stapes and some areas of the hypotympanum cannot be examined. Regular 'second look' operations after 2 years are a must because the recurrence rate is high, especially in cholesteatomas with branching epithelial proliferation. To motivate pa-tients to allow a 'second look' it may be worthwhile postponing the ossicu-lar reconstruction until the second operation. In other words, second stage operations have two purposes – to check for recurrence and to reconstruct the ossicular chain.

Atticotomy with Reconstruction of the Lateral Attic Wall

In cases with a small, sclerosed mastoid, atticotomy is the approach of choice. Removal of the lateral attic wall is easy and the mastoid can be opened if required. If a Schuller's view shows sclerosis of the mastoid, an endaural approach can be used; it is unnecessary to remove a large area of cortical bone to gain access to a small cholesteatoma. It has been shown that it is better to remove the tympanomeatal flap completely and replace it at the end of the procedure than to simply reflect it forward with the consequent risk of traumatising it with the drill and sucker. In this procedure, it is not necessary to remove the cholesteatoma matrix completely; it can be reflected forward while the attic wall is gradually removed (inside-out technique). The bony defect is then closed with a piece of tragal cartilage and perichondrium. The fringe of intact perichondrium helps to keep the cartilage in place. The cholesteatoma matrix is then layed back over the cartilage. Follow-up of many patients has shown that the matrix in its new position acts like normal skin [Plester, 1979].

The technique has similar disadvantages to posterior tympanotomy, i.e. if some squamous epithelium is left behind, it may proliferate and form a cholesteatoma. Another disadvantage is the formation of retraction pockets around the implanted cartilage which may lead to cholesteatoma.

Attico-Antrostomy

Otologists throughout the world unanimously agree that a wide opening between the mastoid cavity and the external auditory canal is the best way to eradicate cholesteatoma. In contrast to the pre-antibiotic era, the classical radical operation is rarely performed, having been largely replaced by a conservative attico-antrostomy preserving the tympanic membrane and ossicles. When should one prefer the open technique and when the closed? The open technique should be used when there is extensive erosion of the attic wall, when there is a labyrinthine fistula or when there is tubal dysfunction. The open technique may also be preferable if there are likely to be difficulties with regular follow-up because the patient comes from a far off place, or in elderly patients, from developing countries.

Attico-antrostomy demands a precise technique and certain points must be observed to avoid complications.

(1) The opening into the canal must be wide enough to allow good aeration and proper drainage. If the entrance to the cavity is narrow, squamous debris will be a constant source of inflammation with infection of the dead cell mass by bacteria and fungi.

(2) All air cells should be smoothed, including the niches and corners in the sino-dural angle, otherwise they may remain a constant source of otorrhoea.

(3) All the bony walls, overhangs and projections must be smoothed with a diamond burr. The facial ridge must be lowered as far as the Fallopian canal. Smooth bony walls help rapid reepithelialisation and prevent the formation of cell debris and granulations. The aim of this technique is to make a small self-cleaning cavity.

Follow-Up

Long-term follow-up by Heumann in children [1983] and by Jahnke et al. in children and adults [pers. communication 1982, 1985] has shown a 30% recurrence rate of cholesteatoma operations after posterior tympanotomy. These figures demonstrate the necessity of a 'second look'. It is important to note, however, that more than half the patients refused a second operation. The high recurrence rate and the low patient compliance make it necessary for the otologist to avoid a posterior tympanotomy without a good doctor-patient relationship. All the facts about the surgery must be explained to the patient and the necessity of two operations must be pointed out. Prior to making a decision about a closed or open technique, consideration must be given to anatomical factors, i.e. pneumatisation of the mastoid, and socio-economic factors, such as the personality and dependability of the patient.

In cases of large cholesteatomas where a cavity is made, the cholesteatoma matrix should be left behind. If the cavity is very large, a split skin graft may be used to line the cavity.

Choice of Surgical Approach and Conclusions

If the patient is young, the mastoid is pneumatised, and if the patient, after a thorough discussion of the possible approaches, understands the necessity of a second look operation 2 years later, a closed technique may be used. In addition, the otologist's personal statistics are obviously much more important than those from other centres. Deguine and Desaulte [1974] in their series found cholesteatoma pearls in 54% of patients.

The fact that cholesteatoma recurs in one-third of the patients and that more than half of the patients, despite thorough precounselling, refuse a second operation has gradually changed the approach in Tübingen in the last 10 years. Clearly, the open technique is preferable. Post-operative evaluation of this procedure certainly shows better results. The recurrence rate dropped to 13.3%, clearly lower than following a closed procedure. Even so, the rate of 13.3% is so high that post-operative follow-up is necessary in every case.

References

Abramson, M.R.G.; Asarch, W.; Litton, B.: Experimental cholesteatoma causing bone resorption. Ann. Otol. *84:* 425 (1975).

Deguine, C.; Desaulte, A.: Traitement du cholestéatome de l'oreille moyenne. Indications de la chirurgie ouverte et fermée. C.r. séanc. 71e Congr. Français d'ORL de Pathologie cervico-faciale, Paris 1974, pp. 181–187.

Gantz, B.J.: Epidermal Langerhans cells in cholesteatoma. Ann. Otol. *93:* 150 (1984).

Heumann, H.: Das Cholesteatom im Kindesalter. Vortrag 67. Vers. der Vereinigung Südwestdeutscher Hals-Nasen-Ohrenärzte, Bamberg 1983.

Heumann, H.; Steinbach, E.: Zur Entstehung des Cholesteatoms als Folge einer experimentell verursachten Mittelohrentzündung. Arch. Otorhinolar. *235:* 577 (1982).

Jahnke, K.; Khatib, M.; Rau, U.: Langzeitergebnisse nach Cholesteatomchirurgie. Lar. Rhinol. Otol. *64:* 238 (1985).

Jansen, C.: Die Erhaltung des äusseren Gehörganges bei der Radikaloperation und eine neue Art der Tympanoplastik. Arch.-Ohr.-Nas.-KehlkHeilk. *182:* 610 (1963).

Lange, W.: Über die Entstehung der Mittelohrcholesteatome. Z. Hals-Nasen-Ohrenheilk. *11:* 250 (1925).

Plester, D.: Chirurgie des Cholesteatoms. Arch. Otorhinolar. *223:* 380 (1979).

Plester, D.; Zöllner, F.: Behandlung der chronischen Mittelohrentzündungen. Hals-Nasen-Ohrenheilkunde in Praxis und Klinik, vol. 6/II (Thieme, Stuttgart 1980).

Poppendieck, J.; Steinbach, E.: Zur granulierenden Myringitis. Arch. Otorhinolar., suppl. II, p. 303 (1983).

Schuknecht, H.F.: Pathology of the ear, p. 218 (Harvard University Press, 1974).

Steinbach, E.: Tierexperimentelle Untersuchungen zur Erzeugung von Cholesteatomen. Laryngol. Rhinol. *57:* 724 (1978).

Steinbach, E.; Grüniger, G.: Experimental production of cholesteatoma in rabbits by using non-irritants. J. Lar. Otol. *94:* 269 (1980).

Prof. Dr. E. Steinbach, Hals-Nasen-Ohrenklinik der Universität Tübingen, Silcherstrasse 5, D–7400 Tübingen (FRG)

Adv. Oto-Rhino-Laryng., vol. 39, pp. 107–110 (Karger, Basel 1988)

Inner Ear Surgery

J. Helms

Department of Otorhinolaryngology, University of Würzburg, Würzburg, FRG

Introduction

Inner ear surgery as a mechanical manipulation at the labyrinthine capsule or in the peri- or endolymphatic space includes obvious risks. Hearing impairment, tinnitus or vestibular dysfunction can be the consequence and is often unavoidable.

Inner Ear Surgery due to Middle Ear and Pyramidal Diseases

During the surgical treatment of the basic disease of an ear it is sometimes impossible to preserve the labyrinthine function. A cholesteatoma with labyrinthitis or a malignant or benign tumor which has grown into the labyrinth, e.g. a glomous tumor, are removed with the labyrinth. If the erosion is less severe the surgeon succeeds in avoiding additional dysfunctions, using a subtile operation technic. This applies mainly for the procedure of labyrinthine fistulas. These fistulas caused by a cholesteatoma are prepared by gradual removal of the detritus and slowly lifting up of the matrix.

If granulation tissue is seen inside the lateral semicircular canal, it is totally removed. Matrix could have grown into the depth. This matrix might be left in place if the perilymphatic space is merely covered and no granulations are present. To avoid post-operative vertigo a mechanically stabile covering is established. After removal of the matrix moist bone paste is applied on top of the fistula. It is additionally covered with fascia or canal skin. Comparing different technics in the treatment of labyrinth

Table I. Inner ear surgery: middle ear and pyramidal diseases

Cholesteatoma with labyrinth fistula	53
Cholesteatoma of the apex of the pyramid	9
Facial neurinoma	6
Mucocele of the apex of the pyramid	4
Arachnoid cyst	4

Table II. Inner ear surgery: diseases of the labyrinth capsule

Stapedectomy	1,210
Stapes revisions	230

fistulas, caused by a cholesteatoma, it was found that this direct covering with bone paste onto the fistula is the most reliable procedure. Post-operative vertigo appeared in 1 of 12 cases where the matrix was preserved in 2 of 14 cases with covering of the fistula using connective tissue and bone, and in 2 of 23 patients with direct bone past apposition. The two vertiginous patients of the last-mentioned group also became symptom-free some weeks after the operation.

All except for 1 patient showed an unimpaired cochlear function. This one ear became deaf, in spite of the fact that the technic was used, which appeared as the most gentle one, namely preserving the matrix (table I).

Diseases of the Labyrinthine Capsule

During stapedectomy only a little part of the procedure, the opening of the foot plate and the insertion of the prosthesis into the vestibulum represents a risk for the inner ear. The complication rate by modern technics is low. Occasionally vertigo and deafness result. Seventy-one of 230 stapes revisions performed in the last 5 years were analyzed. Essentially middle ear problems were encountered. Eleven reossifications in the oval niche, 4 foreign body granulomas, 1 fistula in the oval window close to the prosthesis and 1 otosclerotic obliteration of the round window could be demonstrated as reason for the unsatisfactory results in stapedectomy (table II).

Tumors with Labyrinthine Symptoms

The surgery of acoustic neurinomas is discussed in connection with the inner ear surgery, because inner ear disfunctions may be improved by an early operation. In 30% of patients with an acoustic neurinoma the cochlear nerve could be preserved. The hearing function can only be ensured if the blood supply of the labyrinth supplementary is not permanently harmed during operation. There are considerable uncertainties, because an identification of the important vessels is not reliably possible intraoperatively.

Surgery in Menière's Disease

Inner ear surgery preserving or improving its function is possible in Menière's disease [5] or a partial hydrops of the labyrinth.

The saccotomy [7] represents the logical procedure to reduce an endocochlear hydrops. The surgical manipulation is done a few millimeters away from the sensory organelles. The risks primarily appear low. A saccotomy can only be effective in the case of free patency of the endolymphatic duct. This prerequisite cannot be clarified preoperatively.

The endocochlear shunt operation of Schuknecht [8] is a further operative possibility to preserve the function. A junction between the endo- and perilymphatic space through the round window is formed. Piercing the lamina spiralis ossa it can be ensured that the opening in the high frequency region of the cochlea remains open postoperatively. Six of 17 own patients developed a considerable additional labyrinthine deafness after the operation. These statements are congruent with the experiences of Schuknecht. The procedure seems therefore indicated in cases with severe cochlear lesions.

The results using gentamicin intoxication were not as favourable as those of Lange [6].

As ultima ratio while hearing is worth preserving the transtemporal neurectomy is indicated. In other cases the operation is performed translabyrinthinely [1]. In the histological examination of the excised ganglia vestibulares Scarpae pathologic findings could be seen in light microscopy as well as in electron microscopy. They are published in Helms and Steinbach [4] (light microscopy) and Galic and Helms [2, 3] (electron microscopy) from the ENT Department of the University of Tübingen (table III).

Table III. Inner ear surgery: labyrinth diseases (Ménière's disease, hydrops)

Saccotomy	238
Endocochlear shunt	17
Gentamicin intoxication	10
Transtemporal neurectomy	58
Translabyrinthine neurectomy	79

Discussion

Inner ear surgery is not always destructive when subtile technics are employed. Risks concerning hearing and equilibrium, however, are unavoidable.

References

1   Fisch, U.: Die transtemporale, extralabyrinthäre Chirurgie des inneren Gehörgangs. Arch. klin. exp. Ohr-Hals-Kehlkopfheilk. *194:* 232 (1969).

2   Galic, M.; Helms, J.: Elektronenmikroskopische Untersuchungen über die Häufigkeit, Verteilung und Struktur des Lipofuscins im Ganglion vestibuli bei Morbus Menière. Inserm *68:* 242–262 (1977).

3   Galic, M.; Helms, J.: Elektronenmikroskopische Befunde an Bindegewebe vom Nervus und Ganglion vestibuli bei Morbus Menière. Arch. Otorhinolar. *236:* 67–79 (1982).

4   Helms, J.; Steinbach, E.: Zur pathologischen Anatomie des Morbus Menière. Arch. Ohr.-Nas.-KehlkHeilk. *210:* 357–360 (1974).

5   Helms, J.: Die chirurgische Therapie des Morbus Menière. Arch. Otorhinolar., suppl. I, pp. 67–118 (1985).

6   Lange, G.: Die Indikation zur intratympanalen Gentamycin-Behandlung der Menière'schen Krankheit. HNO *29:* 49–51 (1981).

7   Portmann, G.: The saccus endolymphaticus and on operation for draining the same for the relief of vertigo. J. Lar. Otol. *42:* 809 (1927).

8   Schuknecht, H.F.: Cochleosacculotomy for Menière's disease. Theory, technique, and results. Laryngoscope *92:* 853–858 (1982).

Prof. Dr. J. Helms, Universitäts-Hals-Nasen-Ohren-Klinik, Kopfklinikum, Josef-Schneider-Strasse 11, D–8700 Würzburg (FRG)

Adv. Oto-Rhino-Laryng., vol. 39, pp. 111–119 (Karger, Basel 1988)

Improved Diagnosis of Second Carcinomas by Routine Panendoscopy

J. Poppendieck, M. Schrader

Department of Otorhinolaryngology, University of Tübingen, Tübingen, FRG

The occurrence of double and multiple malignant growths has been reported for many years now [27]. Of almost 20,000 patients with a malignant tumor in the head and neck area in a summarized bibliography compiled by Andrieu-Guitrancourt et al. [1], covering the period 1932 to 1972, 5.9% had a second tumor. Cachin et al. [3], on 5,400 carcinomas of the upper aerodigestive tract, investigated, in particular, the localization of second tumors and established double carcinomas in the same area in 6.1% of cases and double carcinomas in the bronchial system in 0.8% of cases.

The major cause of the statistically higher risk of patients with carcinomas of the upper aerodigestive tract contracting a further tumor in the same area is probably that the exogenic risk factors of tobacco and alcohol abuse are identical for these tumors [5, 9, 21, 22, 30].

The pathogenetic conceptions in this respect were recently reported on by Seitz and Simanowski [23]. Kleinsasser [10] indicates the possibility of an impairment in the immunological tumor defense mechanism in addition to radiogenic second tumors after radiotherapy treatment of the first tumor but only after a dormancy of 20 years on average [10]. He states that only approximately 7–10% of the double carcinomas occur synchronously, but 10% occur within 1 year, a further 30% occur in the 2nd to 5th years and the last third of the second carcinomas do not occur until over 5 years after the first tumor [10].

Assuming that at least those second malignant growths which occur during the first 1–2 years could be localized and co-treated by specific searches as early as the asymptomatic early stage when the first tumor is diagnosed, a number of authors recommend an endoscopic examination of the entire risk area in order to definitively prove the existence or nonexistence of a second tumor [1, 2, 6, 8, 10, 12, 14, 18, 24, 28, 29]. Conversely, Neel [16] rejects such a routine panendoscopy on patients with tumors of the oral cavity, pharynx and larynx, owing to reasons associated with cost effectiveness.

This present study presents the incidence of patients with double tumors at Tübingen University's ENT Department and comments on the question as to whether routine panendoscopy is practical on all patients with a head-neck carcinoma.

Material and Methods

We evaluated the medical records of all patients of our department with a carcinoma of the oral cavity, oropharynx, hypopharynx, esophagus, larynx, trachea or bronchial system, diagnosed between 1980 and 1986. Pretherapeutic panendoscopy was conducted in most cases as from late 1984. This was carried out initially under general anesthesia and artificial respiration with a rigid tube and 0°, 30° and 90° Hopkins optical systems, Karl Storz, Tuttlingen, FRG. Laryngotracheal bronchoscopy, in cases of doubt, in particular for assessing the superior lobe segments, was also carried out with the flexible bronchoscope, inserted through the respiration tube.

After intubation, pharyngo-esophagoscopy was conducted with the optical esophagoscope, Karl Storz, analogously to the procedure implemented by Savary [19], whereby the shoulder and head project beyond the end of the operating table, are held by an assistant and are lowered for inspection of the lower third of the esophagus. After this, a Kleinsasser tube and an operating microscope were used to carefully re-inspect the larynx and, in particular, the hypopharynx, this being the most difficult area to inspect endoscopically. Two percent toluidine blue solution as a vital stain was used as an aid for detecting or determining the spacial extent of tumors, after prior cleaning of the mucous membrane in order to remove saliva, using 1% acetic acid, in particular in the area of the smooth mucous membrane of the esophagus, the pharynx and the floor of the mouth.

The term 'second tumor' was taken to mean a situation in which two mucosal tumors were present, separated by normal mucous membrane which was not stained by toluidine blue and where the pathologist diagnosed an invasively growing carcinoma or at least one carcinoma in situ in each case.

Results

During the period 1980–1986, 712 patients with a total of 755 carcinomas in the area of the oral cavity, oropharynx and hypopharynx, esophagus, larynx, trachea and bronchial system were treated at our clinic. Table I shows a breakdown on the basis of localization and year. This table

Table I. Breakdown of tumors on the basis of localization and year

	1980		1981		1982		1983		1984		1985		1986		1980–1986	
	n	%	n	%	n	%	n	%	n	%	n	%	n	%	n	%
Oral cavity	13	16	20	19	12	13	21	16	9	10	10	10	17	13	102	13
Oropharynx	23	28	33	31	27	29	39	31	26	27	42	43	28	22	218	29
Hypopharynx	9	11	18	18	13	13	15	12	19	20	25	25	30	23	129	17
Oesophagus	6	7	2	1	6	7	2	2	3	3	8	8	7	5	34	5
Larynx supraglottic	6	7	12	12	14	16	18	14	11	12	9	9	13	10	83	11
Larynx glottic, subglottic and panlaryngeal	26	31	22	21	22	24	35	28	28	30	16	15	31	24	180	24
Trachea	–	–	–	–	–	–	–	–	–	–	1	1	1	1	2	0.3
Bronchial system	–	–	–	–	–	–	2	1	1	1	1	1	3	2	7	0.7
Total Tumors	83		107		94		132		97		112		130		755	
Patients	83		101		91		127		94		98		120		712	

The table does not include tumors which occurred before 1980 in patients who developed a second tumor during the observation period; in such cases, only the second tumor is covered in the table. In the case of the other metachronously occurring tumors, both tumors are each recorded in the year of occurrence of the first tumor in order to list each patient once only. As a consequence of the multiple tumors, the sum of the percentages related to localization exceeds 100%.

does not include malignant growths of the facial skin, the salivary glands, the thyroid gland, the nose and paranasal sinuses, the nasopharynx or nonepithelial tumors. It also does not include patients with cervical carcinoma metastases in the case of primary tumors which remained undiscovered. However, panendoscopy was a part of the examination program in such case.

Table II demonstrates how frequently 2 or more tumors were located in the individual years either synchronously or metachronously. It shows the accumulation of synchronous double tumors later than 1984.

Finally, table III covers all tumors of the patients with double or multiple localizations. It can be seen that, by comparison with the accumulation of all 755 tumors in the period 1980–1986 (table I) the oral cavity and oropharynx are clearly overrepresented in the case of the double and multiple tumors. The larynx is clearly underrepresented.

We dispensed with the frequently used designation 'index carcinoma' for the first tumor since, in the case of the synchronous malignant growths, selecting which of the two tumors should be considered as the index carcinoma would frequently have been arbitrary in view of the approximately identical size of the two tumors.

None of the tables allow for 7 bronchial carcinomas which were presumed almost certainly to exist both clinically and radiologically but which, however, were not histologically backed in general owing to a lack of therapeutic consequences in these special cases.

Discussion

The mucous membranes of the upper aerodigestive tract are the organ subjected to the most frequent incidence of multiple carcinomas in the human body [15]. Postmortem examinations indicate that the rate of these multiple tumors is higher than is specified in clinical statistics. Thus, Dargent et al. [7] established double or multiple carcinomas of the esophagus on 30% of patients who had died as the result of ENT tumors, as compared with 5.5% of those who died as a result of other types of tumor. Conversely, the corresponding incidence rates of second tumors in the area of the entire upper aerodigestive tract, reported in retrospective clinical statistics, are only approximately 5% [1, 11]. The vast majority of these tumors were, however, diagnosed metachronously and not synchronously [10, 11]. The

Table II. Synchronous and metachronous diagnosis of double tumors

	Synchronous		Synchronous and metachronous	
	patients	%	patients	%
1980	0	0	5	6
1981	3	3	5	5
1982	2	2.2	6	6.7
1983	2	1.6	7	5.6
1984	2	2.1	6	6.4
1985	9	9.3	14	14.4
1986	7	5.7	10	8.1
1980–1986	25	3.5	53	7.4

The percentages refer to the relevant total number of patients of the year. Patients with metachronously occurring double tumors are listed in the age group of occurrence of the first tumor. Patients whose first tumor occurred before 1980 are listed in the year of the second tumor.

Table III. Localization of all tumors of patients with multiple tumors, synchronous and metachronous

	Syn-chronous	Meta-chronous	Overall		Percentages referred only to the ENT area[1]
			n	%	
Oral cavity	11	9	20	19	23
Oropharynx	21	14	35	33	41
Hypopharynx	10	8	18	17	21
Oesophagus	4	9	13	12	–
Larynx supraglottic	1	4	5	5	6
Larynx glottic	2	6	8	7	9
Bronchial system	2	6	8	7	–
Total	51	56	107	100	100

[1] Not including esophagus or bronchial system.

substantial discrepancy between clinical and postmortem incidence of double tumors can be explained by the fact that the majority of patients with second localizations obviously died as a result of the consequences of the first tumor before the second became symptomatic. Conversely, Martin et al. [13] reported that 20% of their patients suffering from larynx carcinomas and who survived 5 years or more developed a second tumor. Wagenfeld et al. [26] and Wolfensberger and Krause [29] even established that virtually half of all the patients who recovered from their first carcinoma died of a second carcinoma.

High incidence rates of synchronous second tumors were established by the authors who conduct panendoscopy as a routine measure with every tumor of the upper aerodigestive tract, i.e. up to 16% [1, 6, 8, 14, 17, 18].

Most of the multiple tumors which we established synchronously lay in the area of the oral cavity and pharynx. In the case of 4 patients, routine panendoscopy established 5 esophagus carcinomas. In the case of 3 patients, one bronchial carcinoma which, however, was already presumed to exist on the basis of radiological examinations in 2 cases. In 4 patients, there were esophagus carcinomas metachronously at an interval varying between 8 months and 9 years. In 9 patients, there were bronchial carcinomas at intervals varying between 6 months and 6 years.

The clear increase in synchronously discovered carcinomas is striking. We believe that this is largely attributable to the panendoscopy under anesthetic conducted since 1984 in most cases. If, for the period 1984–1986, one only allows for the cases in which panendoscopy was conducted, one obtains an incidence rate of 11.6% in respect of double tumors.

The fact that 12% of the double tumors which occurred synchronously and metachronously lay in the esophagus emphasizes, as does the above-mentioned examination of Dargent et al. [7], the importance of esophago-scopy which, in our opinion, should be carried out with a rigid tube since this is the only safe and reliable method of examining the esophageal orifice. Minor mucosal changes cannot be detected without the use of the Hopkins optical system and air insufflation in particular in the lower esophagus.

Bronchoscopy is subject to the disadvantage that peripheral bronchial carcinomas cannot be detected since the Hopkins optical systems and flexible bronchoscope only permit detection of changes as far as the level of the segmental and sub-segmental bronchea. This fact and also the relatively more seldom incidence of bronchial carcinomas as second tumors in our total test group would make the value of routine bronchoscopy appear questionable.

In addition to the 2 cases of a bronchial carcinoma which were already presumed on the basis of X-ray diagnostics, we found only one unexpected foreign body in the bronchus and, in 1 case only, a bronchus carcinoma synchronously which was not detectable on the X-ray even in retrospect.

Colonna d'Istria et al. [6], McGuirt [14] and Vrabec [25] also report on such tumors which cannot be established by radiological examination and, consequently, they advocate routine bronchoscopy. Conversely, Andrieu-Guitrancourt et al. [1] and Maisel and Vermeersch [12] consider broncho-scopy to be necessary only if radiological examination gives cause to suspect a bronchial carcinoma and if there is a carcinoma of the esophagus, with the aim of establishing any ingrowing in the trachea or bronchial system.

If there is radiological opacity of the lung, one must ask oneself the question as to whether one is dealing with a metastasis of the head and neck tumor or whether there is a bronchial carcinoma as a second tumor. Cahan [4] calculated that there is a 3.5:1 chance of the existence of a bronchial carcinoma as a second tumor in the case of a solitary radiological opacity.

In the case of tumors of the larynx and the hypopharynx, examination under general anesthesia is required for determining the extent and biopsy. Additional bronchoscopy and esophagoscopy during the same anesthetic takes experienced examiners only a few minutes and generally entails no appreciable additional risk to the patient. In the case of tumors of the oral cavity and the oropharynx on which biopsy is conducted under local anes-thetics, such a panendoscopy may be carried out directly before the required tumor operation. We consider the slight extra effort to be justified and practical, both on the basis of reports in the relevant literature and on the basis of our own results, thus giving the attending physician the cer-tainty that he is not treating only one tumor and failing to detect a further tumor. However, should a second tumor be found, the therapeutic concept may be modified accordingly.

We thus consider routine panendoscopy to be one further contribu-tion towards improving the prognosis of our tumor patients. Since, after approximately 2 years, the probability of occurrence of a manifest second tumor becomes greater than that of a recurrence of the first [20], it is advisable to generously interpret the indication for endoscopic examina-tion of the entire risk area even in postoperative care of tumors, in addi-tion to radiological diagnostics.

References

1 Andrieu-Guitrancourt, J.; Brossard-Legrand, M.; Happich, J.L.; Lamy, J.M.: Endoscopie systématique de l'œsophage au cours de cancers buccaux, pharyngés et
laryngés. Ann. Oto-Lar. Chir. cervicofac., Paris *92:* 659–666 (1975).

2 Atkins, J.P.; Keane, W.M.; Young, K.A.; Rowe, L.D.: Value of panendoscopy in
determination of second primary cancer. A study of 451 cases of head and neck
cancer. Archs Otolar. *110:* 533–534 (1984).

3 Cachin, Y.; Luboinski, B.; Schwaab, G.: Association de cancers broncho-pulmo-
naires et de cancers des voies aérodigestives supérieures (43 cas). J. fr. Oto-Rhino-
Lar. *27:* 15–17 (1978).

4 Cahan, W.G.: Lung cancer associated with cancer primary in other sites. Am. J.
Surg. *89:* 494–514 (1955).

5 Castigliano, S.G.: Influence of continued smoking on the incidence of second primary cancers involving mouth, pharynx and larynx. J. Am. dent. Ass. *77:* 580–585
(1968).

6 Colonna d'Istria, J.; Pradoura, J.P.; Zakarian, S.; Jausseran, M.; Musarella, Y.;
Coquin, J.Y.: Les doubles localisations néoplasiques en ORL. Rôle de l'endoscopie.
J. fr. Oto-Rhino-Lar. *29:* 249–256 (1980).

7 Dargent, M.; Noel, P.; Peircula, P.: Etude de la muqueuse œsophagienne au cours de
l'évolution des cancers aérodigestifs supérieurs. J. fr. Oto-Rhino-Lar. *20:* 1089–1092
(1971).

8 Gluckmann, J.L.: Synchronous multiple primary lesions of the upper aerodigestive
system. Archs Otolar. *105:* 597–598 (1979).

9 Greiner, G.F.; Klotz, G.; Conraux, C.; Dillenschneider, E.; Maitre, B.: Les cancers
multiples de la sphère ORL. J. fr. Oto-Rhino-Lar. *18:* 393–395 (1969).

10 Kleinsasser, O.: Bösartige Geschwülste des Kehlkopfes und des Hypopharynx; in
Berendes, Link, Zöllner, Hals- Nasen- Ohren-Heilkunde, vol. 4, part 2, pp. 12.11–
12.13 (Thieme, Stuttgart 1983).

11 Lamprecht, J.; Lamprecht, A.; Morgenstern, C.: Mehrfachtumoren im oberen Aero-
digestivtrakt – eine retrospektive Studie. Laryngol. Rhinol. Otol. *62:* 499–501
(1983).

12 Maisel, R.M.; Vermeersch, H.: Panendoscopy for second primaries in head and neck
cancer. Ann. Oto-Rhino-Lar. *90:* 460–464 (1981).

13 Martin, G.; Glanz, H.; Kleinsasser, O.: Multiple maligne Tumoren bei Patienten mit
Larynxcarcinomen. Lar. Rhinol. Otol. *58:* 756–763 (1979).

14 McGuirt, W.F.: Panendoscopy as a screening examination for simultaneous primary
tumors in head and neck cancer. A prospective sequential study and review of the
literature. Laryngoscope *92:* 569–576 (1982).

15 Mersheimer, W.L.; Ringel, A.; Eisenberg, H.: Some characteristics of multiple primary cancer. Ann. N.Y. Acad. Sci. *114:* 896–921 (1964).

16 Neel, H.B.: Routine panendoscopy. Is it necessary every time? Archs Otolar. *110:*
531–532 (1984).

17 Pasche, R.: Le risque de cancers multiples simultanés ou successifs sur les voies
aérodigestives supérieures chez les porteurs d'un carcinome de la bouche du pharynx
ou du larynx; thèse, Univ. Lausanne (1984).

18   Savary, M.; Crausaz, P.H.; Monnier, P.: La place de l'endoscopie totale aéro-diges-
     tive supérieure en cancérologie. Schweiz. med. Wschr. *109:* 838–840 (1979).
19   Savary, M.; Miller, G.: Der Ösophagus. Lehrbuch und endoskopischer Atlas (Gass-
     mann Verlag, Solothurn 1977).
20   Savary, M.; Pasche, R.; Monnier, P.: Cancer aéro-digestif supérieur: le médecin
     praticien et le médecin spécialiste face au problème du diagnostic précoce. Rev.
     méd. Suisse Romande *99:* 487–497 (1979).
21   Schoenberg, B.S.: Multiple primary neoplasm; in Fraumeni, Persons at high risk of
     cancer (Academic Press, New York 1975).
22   Schottenfeld, D.; Gantt, R.C.; Wynder, E.L.: The role of alcohol and tobacco in
     multiple primary cancers of the upper digestive system, larynx and lung. A prospec-
     tive study. Prev. Med. *3:* 277–293 (1974).
23   Seitz, H.K.; Simanowski, U.A.: Beziehungen zwischen Alkoholkonsum und Krebs-
     erkrankungen. Dt. Ärztebl. *83:* 254–255 (1986).
24   Tucker, H.M.: Cancer of the posterior third of the tongue; in Gates, Current therapy
     in otolaryngology. Head and neck surgery 1984–1985, pp. 223–227 (Mosby, Phila-
     delphia 1984).
25   Vrabec, D.: Multiple primary malignancies of the upper aerodigestive system. Ann.
     Oto-Rhino-Lar. *88:* 846–854 (1979).
26   Wagenfeld, D.J.H.; Harwood, A.R.; Bryce, D.P.; Nostrand, A.W.P.; de Boer, G.:
     Second primary respiratory tract malignant neoplasms in supraglottic carcinoma.
     Archs Otolar. *107:* 135–137 (1981).
27   Warren, S.; Gates, D.: Multiple primary malignant tumors. A survey of the literature
     and a statistical study. Am. J. Cancer *16:* 1358–1414 (1932).
28   Weaver, A.; Flemming, S.M.; Kechtges, T.C.; Smith, D.: Triple endoscopy. A
     neglected essential in head and neck cancer. Surgery *86:* 493–496 (1979).
29   Wolfensberger, M.; Krause, M.: Zur Bedeutung von Fernmetastasen und Zweitkar-
     zinomen als Todesursache bei Patienten mit HNO-Karzinomen. HNO *34:* 296–300
     (1986).
30   Wynder, E.L.; Mushinski, M.H.; Spivak, J.C.: Tobacco and alcohol consumption in
     relation to the development of multiple primary cancers. Cancer *40:* suppl., pp.
     1872–1878 (1977).

Dr. M. Schrader, Hals-Nasen-Ohrenklinik der Universität Tübingen,
Silcherstrasse 5, D–7400 Tübingen (FRG)

Adv. Oto-Rhino-Larying., vol. 39, pp. 120–134 (Karger, Basel 1988)

The Present Status of Surgery in the Treatment of Carcinoma of the Hypopharynx and Cervical Oesophagus

P.M. Stell

Department of Oto-Rhino-Laryngology, Royal Liverpool Hospital, Liverpool, UK

Surgical Anatomy

The hypopharynx is defined by the UICC [1] and the AJC [2] as consisting of three anatomical regions: the postcricoid space, the piriform fossa and the posterior wall of the hypopharynx. The definition of these regions is shown in table I. The lateral limits of the posterior wall of the hypopharynx are not clearly defined by either the UICC or the AJC. They can be defined by an imaginary line prolonged posteriorly from the vocal cords in the cadaveric position; the point where this imaginary line reaches the posterior pharyngeal wall can be regarded as the junction between the lateral wall of the piriform fossa and the posterior pharyngeal wall. Because the same treatment principles apply to tumours of the cervical oesophagus they will also be included in this report.

Surgical Pathology

Histology
All reported cases of hypopharyngeal tumours show that about 95% of these tumours are squamous carcinomas. The author's own series (table II) confirms this.

Site Incidence
The proportions of the author's patients falling into the four anatomical regions are described in table III which shows that just over half the patients had a postcricoid carcinoma. This is a rather unusual distribution,

and there are two reasons for this. Firstly, the author's interest in surgical treatment of postcricoid carcinoma, and, secondly, the fact that within the United Kingdom postcricoid carcinoma remains a relatively common condition whereas in many European countries and North America it is very rare.

Table I. Definition of hypopharynx (AJC/UICC)

1	Pharyngo-esophageal junction (postcricoid area) extends from the level of the arytenoid cartilages and connecting folds to the inferior border of the cricoid cartilage
2	Piriform sinus extends from the pharyngo-epiglottic fold to the upper end of the oesophagus; it is bounded laterally by the thyroid cartilage and medially by the surface of the arytenoepiglottic fold and the arytenoid and cricoid cartilages
3	Posterior pharyngeal wall extends from the level of the floor of the vallecula to the level of the cricoarytenoid joints

Table II. Histological type of tumours

Squamous carcinoma	489
Adenocarcinoma	2
Transitional cell carcinoma	1
Undifferentiated carcinoma	2
Oat cell carcinoma	1
Salivary carcinomas	2
Benign mesodermal tumours	3
Non-Hodgkin's lymphoma	1
Leimyosarcoma	1
Metastatic tumours	1
	503

Table III. Site incidence

Postcricoid space	216
Piriform fossa	194
Posterior wall of hypopharynx	46
Cervical oesophagus	33

Table IV. Lymph node metastases

	N_0	N_1	N_2	N_3	N_X
Postcricoid	124	18	14	21	39
Piriform fossa	55	24	30	50	35
Posterior pharyngeal wall	23	10	2	4	7
Cervical oesophagus	28	0	0	1	4

The N_X category is mainly used for patients previously treated elsewhere.

Table V. T staging of hypopharyngeal tumours (UICC)

Tis	pre-invasive carcinoma (carcinoma in situ)
T0	no evidence of primary tumour
T1	tumour confined to one site
T2	tumour with extension to adjacent site or region without fixation of hemilarynx
T3	tumour with extension to adjacent site or region with fixation of hemilarynx
T4	tumour with extension to bone, cartilage or soft tissues
TX	the minimum requirements to assess the primary tumour cannot be met

Evolution and Spread

It is well known that lymph node metastases are common in piriform fossa tumours and indeed they may be the presenting symptom of this disease. The incidence of lymph node metastases is shown in table IV, using the AJC scheme. A lump in the neck is not always a lymph node metastasis but can be a direct extension of a piriform fossa tumour through the thyroid membrane.

Immobility of the vocal cord is an important event. Its causes include extension of a piriform fossa tumour into the paraglottic space, invasion of the cricoarytenoid joint by either a piriform fossa or a postcricoid tumour, or extension of a postcricoid tumour out of the oesophagus to invade the recurrent laryngeal nerve in the tracheo oesophageal groove.

Postcricoid tumours behave rather like oesophageal tumours and have a fairly wide submucosal spread – on average 1 cm above and below the tumour [3]. Furthermore, they often invade the paratracheal nodes but these nodes are almost never palpable.

The staging of hypopharyngeal tumour by the AJC and UICC schemes is shown in table V. Most of the factors on which this is based are of no practical significance and it would be very much more important to include vocal cord paralysis and the vertical length of a post cricoid tumour (as indeed is done for tumours of the cervical oesophagus). These two factors are the most important prognostic indicators [4].

Invasion of the thyroid gland is also quite common in postcricoid carcinoma rendering attempts to preserve any of the thyroid or parathyroid glands dangerous.

Assessment

Before embarking on surgery it is important to assess the patient very carefully, and as usual this can be divided into five steps: history, clinical examination, laboratory studies, radiology and examination under anaesthesia including biopsy.

The history should include the usual throat symptoms such as dysphagia for food, hoarseness, pain in the ear, etc., but there is only one throat symptom which is relevant to the planning of treatment, and that is hoarseness in a postcricoid carcinoma. This indicates a vocal cord paralysis which in turn usually indicates that the tumour cannot be treated. Of equal importance is enquiry about the patient's previous history and general health: many of these patients are in poor general health, have lost a large amount of weight, many of them smoke and drink heavily and have other intercurrent diseases such as chronic bronchitis, vascular disease, etc. Finally, a small proportion, particularly in the north of England, have a history of irradiation 20–30 years previously, usually for thyrotoxicosis. These patients are exceedingly difficult, and often impossible, to treat.

Clinical examination should pay particular attention to assessing whether a piriform fossa tumour affects both walls of the fossa, how far round the posterior wall the tumour extends, and whether it extends above the pharyngo-epiglottic ligament into the base of the tongue. In both piriform fossa and postcricoid tumours immobility of the vocal cord is an important and frequent sign whose causes have already been described. The patient's neck is examined for lymph node metastases and for mobility of the tumour over the prevertebral fascia. Finally, the patient should have a complete physical examination.

Laboratory investigations often show abnormalities of electrolytes, in particular a low serum potassium, and reduced serum albumin. Again these have an important bearing on treatment and must be corrected as far as possible before surgery is embarked upon.

The standard radiological methods include a lateral soft tissue X-ray of the neck, a barium swallow and a CAT scan. The most informative is often a lateral soft tissue of the neck, certainly in a postcricoid tumour. This almost always shows the upper limit of the tumour clearly, and also its lower limit, if this lies in the neck. If the tumour extends down into the thoracic oesophagus the lower border cannot be seen on a lateral soft tissue of the neck. This is very useful practical information as we wish to know whether the tumour is confined to the neck or whether it extends into the chest. CAT scans are useful for demonstrating invasion of the paratracheal group of lymph nodes within the mediastinum. They do of course show the exact extent of the tumour, although they do not demonstrate cartilage destruction accurately. Data about the exact extent of the tumour might be interesting but usually have little bearing on treatment.

The last and most important step of assessment is examination under anaesthetic which allows a biopsy to be taken. The biopsy is in some ways the least important part of the exercise, and it is more important to assess the extent of the tumour. The essential attributes of piriform fossa tumours which must be assessed before operation include firstly the superior border particularly in relation to the pharyngoepiglottic ligament. About 10% of tumours cross this ligament and invade the base of the tongue: such invasion is easier to palpate with a finger than to see with a laryngoscope. Secondly, it is important to know how far into the posterior pharyngeal wall a piriform fossa tumour extends, since if the tumour extends to the midline of the posterior pharyngeal wall a total pharyngolaryngectomy will be needed. Thirdly, it is important to examine the lower limit of the tumour to ascertain whether it spreads into or lies close to the postcricoid space. If it does then a total pharyngolaryngectomy will be required.

In postcricoid carcinomas we wish to know the level of the upper and lower limits of the tumour. The upper limit can virtually always be seen through an oesophagoscope, and it can be noted whether the tumour extends into the piriform fossa: the latter is important in staging the tumour by the UICC or AJC methods, but has no practical importance whatsoever. The lower limit of the tumour is very important to ascertain but can be quite difficult to find because it is usually not possible to pass an oesophagoscope through a postcricoid tumour. One answer to this problem is to pass a small filiform bougie through the tumour and thread a small bronchoscope, if necessary blind, over the bougie. This manoeuvre will almost always succeed in obtaining access to the oesophagus allowing the lower extent of the tumour to be assessed, and also a feeding tube to be passed if necessary. Again it is necessary to assess the mobility of the tumour over the prevertebral fascia. Finally, a biopsy is taken.

Treatment Policy

It is necessary to consider first those patients who cannot be treated, and then indications for radiotherapy and for surgery. Chemotherapy has so far made no impact whatever on the treatment of hypopharyngeal carcinoma, and will not be considered further.

A very high proportion of patients with hypopharyngeal carcinoma are untreatable – 30% in the author's series. The common causes are very advanced tumour, poor general condition and advanced age, or more commonly combinations of these factors. Distant metastases (2.2%) are a much less common cause of untreatability.

Radiotherapy has little or no part to play in the treatment of piriform fossa tumours. It might have a part to play in small tumours of the posterior pharyngeal wall, but these tumours are so uncommon that it is difficult to make any definite statements about their treatment. It is commonly said that radiotherapy is ineffectual in the treatment of postcricoid carcinoma but this is not true. For 20 years it has been our policy to restrict radiotherapy to those tumours which have a vertical length of less than 5 cm, which have not produced a vocal cord paralysis and which have not metastasised to the lymph nodes in the neck. This treatment policy (fig. 1) produces a 5-year survival of about 30%.

Although radiotherapy is feasible for some patients with small postcricoid tumours the mainstay of management of those hypopharyngeal carcinomas that can be treated is surgery. A very few patients are suitable for partial pharyngectomy and partial laryngectomy (using a modification of the supraglottic laryngectomy technique), and a small proportion of patients with tumours of the posterior pharyngeal wall are suitable for lateral pharyngotomy with preservation of all the larynx. We are therefore concerned mainly with two operations: total laryngectomy plus partial pharyngectomy and total pharyngolaryngectomy. The first of these is possible for piriform fossa tumours only. In the author's experience a partial

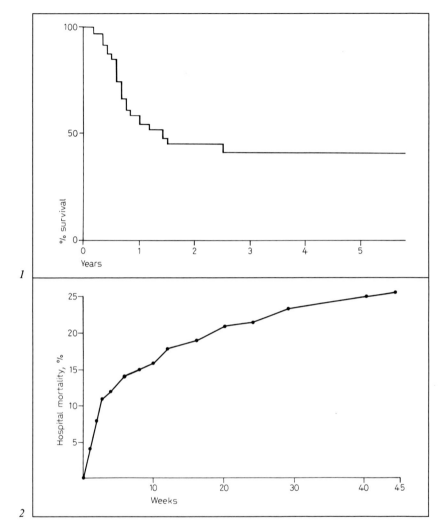

Fig. 1. Survival rate of postcricoid carcinoma treated by radiotherapy.
Fig. 2. Hospital mortality of hypopharyngeal carcinoma.

pharyngectomy (plus of course a total laryngectomy) suffices in 68% of cases. These cases are those where the tumour does not extend into the posterior wall or into the postcricoid space. The remaining 32% require a total pharyngolaryngectomy followed by a pharyngeal reconstruction. Total laryngectomy and partial pharyngectomy needs very little further discussion: it is a similar procedure to that carried out for laryngeal carcinoma and should include removal of one lobe of the thyroid gland. Thyroid and parathyroid replacement is thus not necessary, and the post-operative care is as for a total laryngectomy, except that occasionally dilatation of the repaired pharynx is necessary.

When we turn to postcricoid carcinoma the only feasible procedure is a total pharyngolaryngectomy with resection of a greater or lesser part of the oesophagus. Patients requiring total pharyngolaryngectomy can be divided into 2 categories: firstly those with an extensive piriform fossa tumour or a postcricoid tumour whose inferior border lies 3 cm or more superior to the suprasternal notch, and secondly tumour of the postcricoid space or cervical oesophagus whose lower border lies close to or below the suprasternal notch. The former group need only a total pharyngolaryngectomy whereas the latter group need a total oesophagectomy in addition, and reconstruction thus requires a visceral transplant of pedicled stomach or colon.

Most of the surgical interest now centres on replacement of the pharynx. For many decades this remained one of the unsolved problems of head and neck surgery. Czerny in 1877 performed the first resection of a tumour of the cervical oesophagus, but left the patient with an oesophagostomy and did not attempt to repair the defect. Sporadic attempts were made to repair the cervical oesophagus in the last few years of the 19th century and the first decades of this century, but the first serious attempt to put this operation on a proper footing was made by Wookey of Toronto in 1942 who described an operation in several stages using cervical skin flaps. The whole subject has recently been reviewed thoroughly by Missotten [5] and the following account is based on his work.

Thoracic Skin Flaps

A basic principle in reconstructive surgery is to bring in tissue from another region to remedy a shortage. For the neck the obvious donor area is the chest. Bakamijian revolutionized the whole concept with the introduction of the non-delayed, medially based deltopectoral flap in 1965. This axial pattern skin flap, nourished by branches of the internal mammary artery, very quickly became the method of choice in many centres. Such a flap is raised in one stage outside the irradiated field, it is then rotated, tubed and anastomosed to the stump of the oropharynx under the cervical skin. The remaining fistula is on the chest, thus avoiding any aspiration of saliva. It is closed 3 weeks later.

The deltopectoral flap was a major advance in pharyngoesophageal replacements in the 1960s, but it must be done in at least two stages with a temporary fistula. Furthermore, it does not allow total oesophagectomy and thus might not deal with submucosal spread inferiorly.

The Whole Stomach as a Pedicle Graft

As long ago as 1920, Kirschner pioneered gastric transplantation in a patient with a lye stricture. He brought the stomach to the neck by dividing the left gastric, left gastro-epiploic and short gastric vessels and by tunnelling it subcutaneously. Two years later a gastric pull up was done through the oesophageal bed for carcinoma and it soon became a standard procedure in some centres in the United States even for lesions above the aortic arch.

The rich blood supply, the healing power, and the extreme elasticity of the stomach were first appreciated in 1960 by Ong and Lee who based their new reconstructive method on these properties. They reported 3 gastric transpositions for carcinoma of the pharynx: all 3 patients did well, although the authors admitted that the procedure was formidable, requiring extensive dissection in the neck and opening of both abdominal and thoracic cavities. On the other hand, only a single operation was needed, with only one anastomosis, allowing complete resection of the gullet and resulting in almost perfect degluitition.

The method was refined further by using blind finger dissection and pull-through of the thoracic oesophagus. This procedure had been abandoned for growths of the thoracic oesophagus owing to the dangers arising from adhesions to neighbouring structures, especially the vessels. With a normal thoracic oesophagus these adhesions do not arise, giving the technique the advantage of avoiding a thoracotomy in pharyngeal and cervical oesophageal carcinoma.

Stomach pull up has since become the procedure of choice in various centres, but its success depends largely on the patient's general condition and on the experience of the surgical team. Previous gastric surgery may make this method impossible. Finally, the operation can have unpleasant side effects, such as acid regurgitation or retrosternal discomfort.

A Reversed Gastric Tube

The greater curvature of the stomach can be extensively stretched, thanks to its elasticity and the arrangement of the vessels running in arcades. It is therefore possible to fashion a wide gastric tube attached near the cardiac end and based on the left gastro-epiploic vessels, and to pass it subcutaneously or retrosternally to reach the upper oesophagus.

Advocates of the reversed gastric tube rightly state that its length is adequate and regurgitation oesophagitis minimal. Unfortunately, the extensive closure of the tube and stomach remnant is inevitably fraught with technical difficulties and often severe complications, and this procedure has never been widely used.

Colon as a Pedicle Graft

The colon is an excellent visceral pharyngo-oesophageal substitute with many advantages: its blood supply can be maintained through the marginal artery of Drummond and the vascular arcades. A pharyngocolic anastomosis is unlikely to suffer stenosis. The colonic mucosa has been shown to be relatively resistant to gastric secretions, and, finally, a colonic reconstruction can be performed in one stage.

The first attempts to use large bowel for oesophageal reconstruction were made with transverse colon. Since then many variations have been reported using right, left or transverse colon, in different positions and different peristaltic directions.

In the 1950s, with the appearance of antibiotics and the new bowel preparations, large bowel transposition became an extensively used form of oesophagoplasty. Goligher and Robin popularized colon for pharyngo-esophageal replacement with their two-stage procedure. They mobilized the left colon and brought it through a presternal tunnel to reach from stomach to pharynx.

The retrosternal route has also been advocated, but posterior intrathoracic transplantation is now the procedure of choice, done either under direct vision or blindly with finger dissection and stripping of the oesophagus. The extent of such a procedure, the number of anastomoses and the high risk of leakage are all too often causes of major complications. Despite its many advantages, few centres today use colon transplants, as safer techniques are being developed.

Revascularised Visceral Transplants

Free visceral grafting only became practicable with the advent of microvascular surgery. Seidenberg pioneered this technique for pharyngo-oesophageal reconstruction. He transplanted jejunum to the neck in dogs and anastomosed the mesenteric vessels to the superior thyroid artery and the anterior facial vein. Later this was used in patients.

Various parts of the intestinal tract have been used, including gastric antrum, jejunum, ileum and colon. Most surgeons prefer the upper jejunum because of its accessibility and because its size matches the paryngo-oesophagus.

The reliability of this technique has not yet been confirmed. The bowel does provide an ideal mucosal lined tube, but as for all local procedures, the extent of the resection must be limited. A laparotomy with abdominal anastomoses is necessary, and at least 2 visceral and 2 microvascular anastomoses are needed in the neck, with potential contamination.

Musculocutaneous Claps

In 1896, *La Riforma Medica Napoli* contained a remarkable report by Tansini on reconstruction of the breast with a musculocutaneous latissimus dorsi flap. The flap was based upon blood vessels coming from the underlying muscle. This concept could have had an enormous impact upon reconstructive surgery but Tansini's principle was not recognised.

The musculocutaneous principle was only gradually rediscovered 60–70 years later. Several so-called body units or territories were described, each unit containing a well-defined vascular pedicle, a paddle of muscle and overlying skin in the form of an island.

The main advantages of musculocutaneous flaps are firstly that they can easily be elevated and transferred without delay. Secondly the skin can be doubled over upon itself to form a tube without a fistula, and, thirdly, they can provide a large amount of well vascularised tissue for an irradiated, ischaemic or infected area. Their disadvantages, seemingly few, are that they are bulky, adynamic and often insensitive, and leave a large donor defect.

The pectoralis major flap was pioneered by Ariyan in 1979 and since then it has become the skin flap of choice in pharyngo-oesophageal reconstruction pushing the delto-pectoral flap into second place. The latissimus dorsi flap has occasionally served the same purpose.

Miscellaneous Methods

Free skin grafting has been tried but has now been largely abandoned, as have laryngotracheal autografts and local mucosal flaps.

Foreign Material

Interesting results have occasionally been reported on the use of lypo-hilized aorta to secure continuity between the pharynx and oesophagus in animals, but vascular homo- or heterografts have been tried experimentally many more times with very little success, because they often lead to strictures and fistulae.

Reconstruction by plastic tubes has been used temporarily between stages of cervical reconstruction to: (a) eliminate salivary leakage; (b) direct the saliva into the stomach; (c) maintain a widely patent oesophagus and pharynx, and (d) create a trough between them.

Permanent plastic tubes in the neck were first advocated by Stuart for repair after potentially curative resections, especially in poor risk patients, or as a palliation for inoperable carcinomas.

Neck Nodes

The proportion of patients with a hypopharyngeal carcinoma, who have neck nodes at presentation vary from 3% for tumours of the cervical oesophagus to 65% for piriform fossa tumours. Patients with lymph nodes at presentation were treated in the present series by radical neck dissection, but prophylactic or functional neck dissection was not used.

Results

The present account is based on the author's experience of 177 pharyngeal replacements carried out in the last 24 years. The main method for replacement after total pharyngo-oesophagectomy has been gastric transposition; after pharyngolaryngectomy for more limited tumours the delto-pectoral flap was used from 1965 to 1980, then the pectoralis major flap from 1980 to 1984, and, finally, the revascularised ileal loop for the past 2 years.

Survival

Survival curves for the various forms of repair are shown in figure 3, which shows that a 5-year acturarial survival of about 30% can be achieved with each method. However, it is not justifiable to compare these curves with each other because the underlying patient population is different.

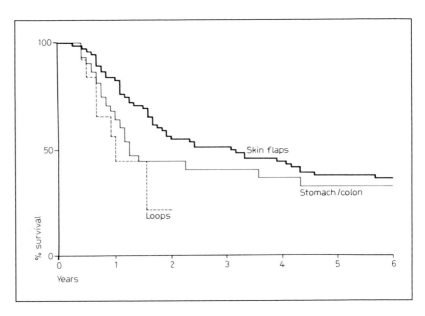

Fig. 3. Hypopharynx reconstruction. Actuarial survival after various different forms
of repair.

Mortality

Total pharyngolaryngectomy is the head and neck operation par excellence which can cause the death of the patient. This indeed is one of the main criteria when judging the various methods of replacing the hypopharynx, but sadly there is no standard method of reporting mortality. Some surgeons report deaths during the operation, some within 24 h, some within 1 week and some before the patient leaves hospital healed and swallowing. It is thus possible to claim a mortality ranging from 1 to 25 % depending upon the time interval chosen (as is shown in figure 2 based on the author's own material). Figures for intercurrent deaths within 7 days, intercurrent deaths after 7 days and death from cancer before the patient is completely healed, are shown in table VIII for the various forms of repair. This table shows that including deaths within 7 days, a standard period which is often used, misses 62 % of the surgical deaths in patients undergoing gastric transposition. Skin flap repair has a high long-term *hospital* mortality due to late events such as death from lung abscess or from recurrent cancer before healing is complete.

Table VI. Median stay in hospital (days)

Skin flaps	82
Stomach/colon	37
Revascularised loops	21

Table VII. Incidence of stenosis

	Total number at risk	Number	%
Stomach/colon	31	31	3
Skin flaps	86	33	38
Revascularised loops	17	2	2

Table VIII. Hospital mortality

	Total	Death from ICD		Death from cancer before healing complete	Total	
		within 7 days	after 7 days		n	%
Stomach/colon	53	7	14	1	22	42
Skin flaps	105	0	12	7	19	18
Revascularised flaps	19	0	2	0	· 2	11

Morbidity

The most important parameters of morbidity are stricture formation and length of stay in hospital. These are shown for the author's own material in tables VI and VII. It can be seen that the use of skin flaps requires a long stay in hospital and has a high incidence of stricture formation, that is patients require one or more dilatations of the pharynx.

The causes of long-term morbidity after discharge from hospital also include the necessity to administer substitution therapy for the thyroid and para-thyroid glands in patients who have undergone total pharyngolaryngectomy, and in the great difficulty in learning any form of replacement speech. Fewer than 10% of these patients learn 'oesophageal' speech, and the only satisfactory solution at the moment appears to be one of the hand-held devices but these produce a rather mechanical sounding and not very serviceable voice. The more recent techniques of tracheopharyngeal shunt do not appear to be of any benefit in this disease.

References

1   UICC: TNM classification of malignant tumours, pp. 18–19 (UICC, Geneva 1978).
2   American Joint Committee for Cancer Staging and End Result Reporting: Manual for staging of cancer (Chicago 1977).
3   Harrison, D.F.N.: Pathology of hypopharyngeal cancer in relation to surgical management. J. Lar. *84:* 349–367 (1970).
4   Willatt, D.J.; Jackson, S.R.; McCormick, M.S.; Lubsen, H.; Michaels, L.; Stell, P.M.: Vocal cord paralysis and tumour length in staging postcricoid cancer. Eur. J. Surgi. Oncol. *13:* 131–140 (1987).
5   Missotten, F.E.M.: Review. Historical review of pharyngo-oesophageal reconstruction after resection for carcinoma of pharynx and cervical oesophagus. Clin. Otolar. *8:* 345–362 (1983).

P.M. Stell, ChM, FRCS, Department of Oto-Rhino-Laryngology,
Royal Liverpool Hospital, Prescot Street, P.O. Box 147, Liverpool L69 3BX (UK)

Adv. Oto-Rhino-Laryng., vol. 39, pp. 135–144 (Karger, Basel 1988)

Experience in Endoscopic Laser Surgery of Malignant Tumours of the Upper Aero-Digestive Tract

W. Steiner

Department of Otorhinolaryngology, University of Göttingen, Göttingen, FRG

The following report is based on the author's personal experience regarding the possibilities for application of laser surgery in the treatment of malignant tumours of the upper aero-digestive tract. Examples taken from different organs are presented to show the possibilities and limitations of palliative-symptomatic and curative mono- and combination therapy. Between 1979 and 1986, the author treated almost 900 cancer patients, using laser surgery, and his experience, mainly with laryngeal carcinoma (more than 500 patients) is presented here.

Palliative-Symptomatic Laser Therapy

There can be no doubt about the progress made by the application of laser surgery in the symptomatic-palliative treatment of far-advanced, inoperable and/or incurable primary or recurrent tumours or metastases deriving from other organs. In these cases it is the aim of endoscopic-microsurgical laser therapy to remove, as far as possible, the tumour stenosis responsible for the impairment of breathing or swallowing (fig. 1).

We prefer the argon laser for treatment of the nasopharynx and trachea. In most cases tracheotomy can be avoided by the extensive vaporization of the stenosing tumour in the region of the upper airways, and thus the suffering of the patients with hopeless prognosis can be relieved.

The CO_2 laser with microscope is employed in the en- and transoral laser surgical treatment of malignant tumours in the oro- and hypopharynx and in the larynx. This kind of laser surgery is difficult and the ability to

correctly estimate the size of the area to be resected is acquired by experience, according to the principle 'not too much and not too little'. It would
be a grave misunderstanding to assume that this is a 'surgery for beginners'
learning the basics of laser surgery. A misunderstanding like this would be
definitely harmful to the patient.

Laser-Microsurgery of the Laryngeal Carcinoma –
Curative Monotherapy for Early Stages

Larynx ($_pT_{is}$, $_pT_1$, $_pT_{2'small'}$ vocal cord mobile)
Since 1975 we have favoured the endoscopic treatment of early cancer
stages in the larynx, and since 1979 we have been using the CO_2 laser.

The main advantage of transoral microscopically controlled, virtually
bloodless laser surgery is the possibility of reliably excising the tumour in
a manner that complies with onco-surgical requirements, while preserving a maximum of function. Our experience to date suggests that this surgical approach is the more preferable method. With adequate exposure of
the tumour-bearing endolarynx, microlaryngoscopic resection for the
treatment of early cancer stages is a sparing procedure, which can often
be performed on an outpatient basis, and is not associated with major
side effects or complications. The resection may be reliably performed
without need of a tracheotomy, because of the lack of severe post-operative oedema.

The decisive statement with regard to oncology is the fact that until
1986 only 1 patient had to be laryngectomized, and that not a single
patient with an early stage of cancer of the larynx died from his laryngeal
growth.

Indications. In early stages of cancer of the glottis and the supraglottis,
removal of the tumour within healthy tissue can normally be controlled by
histological examination. The circumscribed carcinoma in situ or carcinoma limited to the middle of the freely mobile vocal cord represents the
ideal indication for endolaryngeal microsurgical resection, even without
laser. In these cases, the tumour can be excised in every direction with a
margin of healthy tissue. The ideal case, as hoped for by the laryngeal
surgeon and the pathologist, is when the distance between the tumour and
the coagulation line is so large that an 'assessment zone' for patho-histo-
logical examination is present.

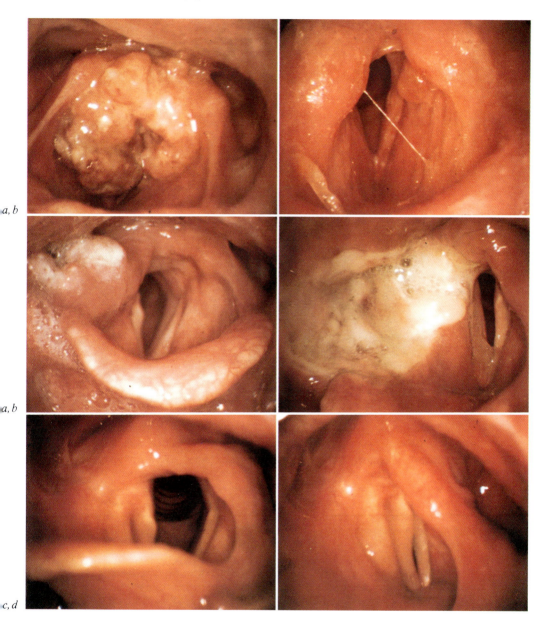

a, b

a, b

c, d

Fig. 1. Extensive carcinoma of the larynx in a 91-year-old patient. *a* Findings before a laser-surgical symptomatic-palliative debulking of the tumour because of severe apnea. Microlaryngoscopic laser-surgical treatment as an alternative to a tracheotomy. *b* Circumscribed residual tumour in the area of the left arytenoid cartilage 1 year after laser-surgical resection and radiotherapy, which could be started because of the generally good condition. The recurrence of the tumour was again microlaryngoscopically removed with the laser. The patient died from heart failure at the age of 93 without any clinical indication for a local recurrence of the tumour.

Fig. 2. Hypopharyngeal carcinoma on the right side (pT_2, pN_oM_x) 68-year-old male. Microlaryngoscopic laser resection and elective regional functional neck dissection on the right side (6/82) (no tracheotomy, stomach tube: 4 days; period of hospitalization: 8 days). Local-regional absence of a recurrence for almost 5 years now. *a* Pre-therapeutic findings. *b* 10th post-operative day: fibrin deposits in the area of the resection. *c* Post-therapeutic findings during inspiration. *d* Post-therapeutic findings during phonation. Organic functional result constant for the last 5 years: respiratory function normal, vocal function very good, swallowing function unimpaired. The pre- and post-therapeutic findings were documented with the Wolf magnifying laryngopharyngoscope.

Borderline Indications. In the case of more extensive growth of the vocal cords, the histological evaluation of the marginal zone may be difficult. This applies particularly to carcinomas of the vocal cord that have reached the anterior commissure, and/or extend far into Morgagni's ventricle and/or are spreading subglottically. Resection in these cases extends up to the thyroid, arytenoid or cricoid cartilage.

Larynx ($_pT_{2'large}$, vocal cord mobility impaired,

$_pT_{3\ without\ fixation}$, $_pT_{4\ circumscribed}$)

Increasing experience with the use of microscopically controlled laser surgery within the larynx has also shown that 'advanced T_2 tumours', T_3 tumours 'without fixation', and 'circumscribed T_4' tumours can be successfully treated, curatively, with microlaryngoscopic laser surgery. The patients concerned adamantly refused external-approach surgery, insisting instead on endoscopic laser surgery, and eventually did not even permit oncologically indicated post-operative irradiation of the primary tumour and the neck.

In the case of these tumours, endoscopic treatment competed with the classical vertical and horizontal partial resections which in certain cases may mean more oncological safety, especially by the excision of the cartilage next to the tumour performed in each case. An intra-operative changeover from endolaryngeal to extralaryngeal partial resection is readily possible at any time, if, for example, it proves impossible to expose the tumour region adequately. Tumour involvement of the pre-epiglottic space – whether diagnosed pre-operatively or intra-operatively – or tumour invasion of the oropharynx and/or hypopharynx, or involvement of an arytenoid cartilage, do not set limitations on the transoral microsurgical procedure. Borderline indications are marked subglottic spread, and involvement of the entire inter-arytenoid region.

Contraindications. The *limits* of the endolaryngeal laser-surgical approach are reached whenever the carcinoma has spread beyond the larynx, that is, the tumour has 'broken out' from between the cricoid and thyroid cartilages. This also applies in the case of growth into the cricoid over a wide front, and involvement of both arytenoid cartilages.

Unfortunately, despite the advances made in the field of diagnostic radiology, tumour infiltration and spread cannot always be reliably detected in the pre-treatment phase – not even with computerized tomography.

Treatment of Early Cancer Stages by Laser Microsurgery:
Oral Cavity, Oro-Hypopharynx

En- or transoral laser resection is performed in patients with primary tumours in the oral cavity as well as in the oro- and hypopharynx, if these growths, as judged by their location and extension, are regarded as operable by partial resection with preservation of organ integrity and function, and if according to the overall oncological situation there is a chance for success of a curative therapy. Post-operative radiotherapy may be dispensed with after removal of the primary tumour with a wide safety margin and after regional functional neck dissection, if metastases can be excluded ($_pN_0$) by histological verification, or if only a small, solitary (micro-) metastasis ($_pN_1$) remains. By not closing the defects after enoral laser resection of malignant tumours, excellent final healing results with largely preserved function may be attained, even in the case of large wound cavities (fig. 2).

Since we are only rarely confronted with a truly osseous, histologically verified tumour infiltration, it is in most instances sufficient to perform resection along the bone, if necessary with removal of the periosteum. The moderate disadvantages (by not performing primary defect closure) such as foetor development due to necroses and light post-operative bleeding, are largely avoided by temporary sutures (for about 5 days) to reduce the size of the wound. In view of the definitive advantages of better functional rehabilitation and easier early recognition of recurrences, these small disadvantages are of little concern. On the basis of the follow-up experience gained up to now it seems justified to abstain from block resection. Oncologically, the results are comparable to those of conventional surgery.

Curative Combined Therapy (laser surgery and postoperative irradiation) for Very Advanced Laryngeal Tumours, instead of Total Laryngectomy

Larynx (large 'T₃ with fixation', 'advanced T₄')

Since the early 1980s we have removed advanced laryngeal carcinomas by transoral microlaryngoscopic laser surgery whereby we preserve, as far as possible, functionally important organ structures, and employed post-operative radiotherapy with the aim to spare the patient a laryngectomy.

In cases of T_3 tumours with fixation, and advanced T_4 tumours that are too extensive and/or too unfavourably located for partial resection, we prefer a combined therapy comprising laser surgery and postoperative irradiation, as an alternative to the total laryngectomy, which, in any case, should always be at the bottom of the list of surgical measures aimed at preserving function. Here, the tumour mass is microlaryngoscopically resected with the laser, or debulked to the extent that, with laryngopharyngeal functions preserved or restored, the biological prerequisites for postoperative treatment in the form of, for example, radiotherapy, are improved.

It has been seen that even extensive resections can often be performed without tracheotomy. Large areas of cartilage in the thyroid, cricoid and arytenoid regions are exposed, coagulated and, where necessary, removed. Irradiation can be started after 2 weeks, without having to fear such complications as oedema or perichondritis. The oncological and functional results so far achieved, justify the pursuance of this therapeutic concept.

New Concepts for the Therapy of Advanced Tumours: Laser Surgery and Post-Operative Radiotherapy

Abandoning Block Resection and Defect Closure: Justification and Consequences

For exactly 10 years now, our policy has been: to abandon radical, mutilating surgery of the head and neck with its only minimal improvement of life expectancy, in favour of function-preserving therapy that improves the quality of the patient's life. This has been accomplished by extended, modified classical partial laryngectomies and by function-preserving surgery of the cervical lymph system. In the meantime, this approach has been decisively aided by the new possibilities of being able to surgically remove even advanced tumours of the oral cavity, pharynx and larynx enorally and/or transorally, using the CO_2 laser under microscopic control.

With this approach, involving the separate surgical treatment of the primary tumour and the neck, we turned our backs on the two internationally recognized oncosurgical principles of block resection and defect closure with skin-muscle flaps or grafts.

The first of these two principles can be refuted only on the basis of a long-term follow-up of representative case material, comparable to the other groups, but our observations and results to date clearly indicate that this approach should definitely be pursued further. In the case of the second principle, a whole series of arguments can already be presented in favour of dispensing with primary closure of the defect.

As a result of abandoning primary defect closure, the early detection of recurrent lesions is facilitated, and very good definitive wound healing is achieved with maximum preservation of function, even in the case of large wound cavities. When the filling of the defect with granulation tissue and re-epithelialization has been completed – within 6–8 weeks – the results of wound healing in terms of the restitution of normal breathing, swallowing and speech, are usually highly satisfactory.

Only rarely does a tracheotomy become necessary. In comparison with conventional surgical techniques employing flaps to cover the defect, the in situ duration of the gastric tube is appreciably shorter, as is also the postoperative period of hospitalization. By dispensing with block resection and closure of the defect, the complication rate has also been reduced. Fistulas between the treated primary tumour and the neck are very rarely observed, since, as a rule, an adequately thick layer of tissue can be preserved, as a sort of sealing material. If, during laser resection of the primary tumour, it becomes clear that, for anatomical-oncological and/or surgical-technical reasons, the procedure is not going to succeed, a neck dissection, performed 4–6 days later, is recommended.

In recent years, we have – for oncobiological reasons – gone over to allowing a certain time to elapse between resection of the primary tumour and the subsequent neck dissection.

Finally, another advantage might be mentioned. Only 2 weeks following surgical laser treatment, irradiation can be started, wherever it is indicated for oncological reasons.

How can we justify this understandably still controversial new concept – involving the abandonment of block resection on the one hand and debulking of advanced tumours with subsequent radiotherapy and/or chemotherapy on the other, and whose aim is to preserve functionally important organ structures, as an alternative to mutilating surgery?

Reflections on this must be seen against the background of generally very unfavourable survival times of patients with advanced carcinomas of the upper aero-digestive tract.

Despite aggressive combination therapy – which usually also involves radical, mutilating surgery of the primary tumour and, for example, in advanced tumours of the larynx, hypopharynx and base of the tongue, also a laryngectomy, partial resection of the pharynx or complete pharyngectomy with radical neck dissection and postoperative radiation treatment – the prognosis for these patients has not significantly improved over the last decades.

We all know that the fate of the patient with carcinoma of the upper aero-digestive tract is relatively seldom decided by the nature of the treatment of the primary tumour. The proponents of the conventional treatment concept are guided by the idea of appreciably improving the patient's chances of surviving, or of even being able to cure him, by submitting the primary tumour to super-radical treatment. Apparently, however, they are overlooking the fact that the most common causes of death are advanced neck metastases, distant metastases, or secondary carcinomas in the oesophagus or bronchi, which are not surgically manageable.

Advanced age, poor nutritional status and a generally reduced state of health, together with severe underlying cardiac, pulmonary and hepatic disease (often due to smoking and drinking – the major aetiological factors for the development of cancer) represent additional factors limiting the patient's life expectancy.

Side Effects/Complications

Side effects and complications arising in laser surgery of malignant tumours of the upper aero-digestive tract are largely determined by the kind of artificial respiration employed (intubation, jet ventilation), by location and extent of the resection, and by kind and dose of previous radiotherapy. Post-operative bleeding, respiratory distress, aspiration, skin emphysema, secondary cicatricial stenoses, etc. cannot be regarded as typical complications of laser treatment since they are also observed (even more frequently) in conventional tumour surgery.

In two of several thousand endolaryngeal microsurgical laser operations, endotracheal tube fires occurred due to insufficient covering with moist gauze. There were no definitive organic or functional consequences for the patients.

Advantages of Laser Surgery

The main advantage is the absence of any direct contact during surgery which results in only very little bleeding and provides a dry field of operation and precise preparation layer by layer. Owing to the improved view and to the enlargement of the field of vision, the tumour can be resected in an oncologically reliable way, with a maximum preservation of tissue.

Healthy, tumour-free and functionally important organ structures can be better preserved than by any other classical partial external resection, however perfectly it may be performed.

The haemostatic effect of the laser during surgery, together with concomitant conventional coagulation of larger vessels, serves not only to improve vision and enable more precise resection, but also checks bleeding quite substantially. Further advantages are the absence or only moderate rate of complications like perichondritis or post-operative oedema, rendering a tracheotomy unnecessary even in more extended resections. The time required for operation and the postoperative period of hospitalization are thus shortened appreciably.

There are further observations and considerations that are connected with laser surgery, such as sterilization of the operative field with regard to tumour cells and bacteria as well as the prevention of mechanical spreading of tumour cells and the sealing of lymph vessels which quite possibly helps to prevent lymphogenic metastasis formation.

Finally, the patient profits in yet another way from laser treatment. Unlike radiotherapy, laser surgery may be repeated at any time if recurrences arise. If necessary, subsequent surgical, radio- or chemotherapeutic treatment can be applied without disadvantages to the patient and without the fear of complications.

Prerequisites of Laser Surgery of Malignant Tumours

Prerequisites for the successful application of microlaryngoscopic surgical laser techniques in the treatment of malignant tumours are: (1) Experience on the part of the therapist with conventional tumour surgery, endolaryngeal microsurgery, and laser surgery. (2) Optimal exposure of the region affected by the tumour. (3) Close cooperation with an experienced pathologist. (4) Intensive follow-up. (5) Cooperation of the informed patient.

To ensure complete tumour removal, consecutive samples of resected tumour and marginal tissue must be closely studied, and intra-operatively histological examination of immediate sections may be necessary.

Before carrying out surgery, the patient should be properly informed about the 'stepwise approach' in the sense of 'customized surgery', and about the possible need for an immediate or subsequently more radical intervention. The stepwise approach offers the patient the greatest chance of preserving the functionally important structures of the larynx, while, at the same time, guaranteeing a high degree of oncological safety.

The conditions I have just mentioned indicate that we are not concerned here with routine 'everyday surgery', which is indeed not suitable for 'everyone'.

Conclusions

The possibilities for application of various laser systems (CO_2, argon) in endoscopy-supported and microscope-controlled treatment of malignant tumours of the upper aero-digestive tract have opened up a new therapeutic dimension. Between 1979 and 1986, the author treated almost 900 cancer patients (15–91 years old), using laser surgery. His experience with laryngeal carcinoma (more than 500 patients) is primarily presented here to illustrate the possibilities and limitations of laser surgery.

In the early stages of growth, transoral microsurgical resection using the CO_2 laser as curative monotherapy, is the preferred method. The great advantage of this procedure is its high, virtually bloodless, precision in the removal of the tumour, which makes it oncologically reliable, while permitting satisfactory functional results.

The decisive advance brought by laser surgery is the possibility of being able to treat, transorally, even advanced tumours palliative-symptomatically or curatively – alone or in combination with radiotherapy, while preserving functionally important organ structures – often without need of a tracheotomy. Dispensing with block resection and defect closure would seem justified.

Prerequisites for the successful application of laser surgery – which is certainly not 'surgery for everyone' and not equally suitable for all patients alike – include close cooperation with an experienced pathologist, and meticulous follow-up examinations.

Long-term observations will show what the future potentialities and limits of laser surgery are, and what its final value will prove to be, within the framework of combined therapeutic procedures.

References

Steiner, W.: Aspects of clinical differential diagnosis and therapy of early laryngeal cancer (microcarcinoma). Clinics in oncology, vol. 1, No. 2 (Saunders, Philadelphia 1982).

Steiner, W.: Endoscopic therapy of early laryngeal cancer, indications and results; in Wigand, Steiner, Stell, Functional partial laryngectomy, conservation surgery for carcinoma of the larynx, p. 163 (Springer, Berlin 1984).

Steiner, W.: Endoskopische und mikroskopische Laser-Chirurgie im oberen Aero-Digestivtrakt; in Buess, Unz, Pichlmaier, Endoskopische Techniken, p. 150 (Deutscher Ärzteverlag, Köln 1984).

Steiner, W.: Einsatzmöglichkeiten von Lasern im Bereich des oberen Aero-Digestivtraktes. Laser Med. Surg. 2: 75 (1986).

Steiner, W.; Herbst, M.: Kombinationsbehandlung von Hypopharynxkarzinomen mit endoskopischer Laserchirurgie und Nachbestrahlung, in Sauer, Kombinationstherapie der Oropharynx- und Hypopharynxkarzinome. Sonderbände zur Strahlentherapie und Onkologie, vol. 91, p. 108 (Urban & Schwarzenberg, München 1987).

Prof. Dr. W. Steiner, Universitäts-Hals-Nasen-Ohrenklinik,
Robert-Koch-Strasse 40, D–3400 Göttingen (FRG)

Adv. Oto-Rhino-Laryng., vol. 39, pp. 145–147 (Karger, Basel 1988)

Our Concepts of Management of Lower Alveolar Sulcus Carcinoma

A. Pusalkar

Department of Otolaryngology, T.N. Medical College and B.Y.L. Nair Hospital (Head: Prof. Dr. *A.G. Pusalkar*), Bombay, India

Anatomically, alveolous is formed by the alveolar process of maxilla and the mandibule. The alveolar sulcus is the region lateral to the mandibular alveolar process called the lower alveolar sulcus. This sulcus is formed by the mucosal fold which runs from the mandibular process to the cheek. The management of tumours in this area largely depends on the location of the tumour in the sulcus. Broadly, this region can be divided into three zones: anterior, middle and posterior. The tumours which had crossed the mandible medially involving sublingual sulcus or crossed retromolar trigone medially to the tonsils or the palate are omitted.

Forty percent of cancers in India are in the head and neck region, and 25% of these are localised to the lower alveolar sulcus. In addition to malnutrition, and poor dental hygiene by far the single most important cause which predisposes to malignancy in this region is tobacco chewing.

The habit of eating betal leaf ('paan' as it is called) is an age-old custom in India. This leaf, along with some perfumed ingredients, is offered to the guests as a mark of respect. It is quite common to eat it after dinner or a good meal. The basic ingredients are quite harmless and contain mild astringent agents which help the digestion.

This harmless custom became dangerous only after tobacco came to India about 500 years ago. Over the subsequent years, the harmless ingredients were replaced by calcium hydroxide – which is a strong alkali – and tobacco. There are some sections of the people who make a small ball of mixture of tobacco and calcium hydroxide and keep it in alveolar sulcus. The mixture remains in place for 8–12 h a day. Ninety-eight percent of people with carcinoma of this region are habitual tobacco chewers. The site of malignancy is always specific to the site where this mixture is kept. Calcium hydroxide causes superficial burns of the oral mucosa and tobacco acts on the area, and, over the years, leucoplakia of various different types develop followed by malignancy. In the last 8 years the total number of head and neck tumours treated in our department were 1,562. Of these, 420 were tumours in the lower alveolar sulcus.

As we have just seen for classification purpose, this region can be divided into three zones, anterior, middle and retromolar, and the extent can be classified as superficial, deep with involvement of skin, and deep with infiltration of pterygopalatine fossa.

By the time majority of the patients come for medical help the tumour has already reached an advanced stage of malignancy. This is due to inadequate medical facilities in villages and ignorance on the part of the patient. Unfortunately, pain is not a predominant symptom at the initial stage. Due to such an advanced nature of the tumours management becomes difficult. Malnutrition, hypoproteinemia, and poor general condition add further to the problem of management.

Even though surgical excision of large-sized tumours is possible in this region, adequate reconstruction with maintenance of physiological function becomes a major problem. Thus, aims of management would be: eradication of the disease; restoration of legible speech and swollowing; aesthetically acceptable and results; cost factor?

All 420 patients which are being presented underwent primarily surgical management followed by radiation. Chemotherapy was an adjuvant therapy in some. In all 420 cases, radical neck dissection was performed simultaneously irrespective of palpable or otherwise lymph nodes. Seventeen cases with severe trismus received chemotherapy.

Till about 2½ years ago, irrespective of the size or site of tumour, surgical management consisted of hemimandibulectomy with local soft tissue reconstruction. Hemimandibulectomy is done with excision of the condyle. The pterygoid muscles are preserved and sutured. The cheek mucosa is sutured to the edge of the tongue, for inner lining.

This surgical method is quick. Though aesthetically the end result may not be satisfactory, functionally the patients are quite satisfied.

When the tumours involved the skin, the large defects were reconstructed in staged procedures. The two common flaps were the deltopectoral flap and the forehead flap. This caused many days of hospitalisation sometimes up to 3 months and due to poor general condition in some patients the deltopectoral flap would fail causing further delay. The forehead flap is a very vascular flap and almost never fails but leaves a very large defect and scar on the forehead.

For the last 2½ years we have a slightly different approach. We try to avoid hemimandibulectomy with removal of condyle, as it causes profuse bleeding from the pterygoid plexus and we feel it is not necessary.

If the tumours are superficial, a $T_1 T_2$ horizontal wedge is removed with the tumour and the cheek mucosa is sutured to the sublingual mucosa. If the tumours are large without involvement of skin, partial mandibulectomy is done and the defect is closed as local soft tissue mucosal lining or the bony gap is bridged with free iliac crest.

All the large defects caused after excision of infiltrated skin are bridged now by the pectoralis major myocutaneous or osteomyocutaneous flap. This is the most versatile flap. In the last 3 years we have done 69 pectoralis major myocutaneous flaps and 18 osteomyocutaneous flaps. Not a single skin graft of the flap has failed. We are, however, a bit sceptical about the osteomyocutaneous flap because out of 18 flaps 6 ribs got necrosed and had to be removed.

If we look at the overall results of management of such large tumours there are two groups of patients, one with superficial tumours, and the second with deep tumours with skin involvement. And for each group there are two distinct modes of surgical management. Superficial tumors are radically managed with hemimandibulectomy and soft tissue reconstruction. And deep tumours with skin involvement are managed by partial mandibulectomy with iliac crest reconstruction of the mandible.

Advanced tumours are also managed in two different ways, in one group radically excised and reconstructed in two stages and in the other group radically excised but primarily reconstructed with pectoralis major/osteomyocutaneous flap. For both I have a follow-up of 5 and 2½ years for comparison of our aims of management. Only general terminology such as fair, good and poor is used.

I would like to conclude by saying that I personally feel the best way to reconstruct such large defects would be to use free flaps with the microvascular technique. I have attempted only one reconstruction with this technique which was partially successful. But I am convinced that microvascular free flaps would be the final answer for reconstructing these defects.

Prof. Dr. A.G. Pusalkar, Department of Otolaryngology,
T.N. Medical College and B.Y.L. Nair Hospital, Bombay (India)

Subject Index